T0134342

POCKET GUIDE FOR CUTANEOUS MEDICINE AND SURGERY

The *Pocket Guide for Cutaneous Medicine and Surgery* is written for dermatology residents and clerkship students. It contains up-to-date and easily accessible medical and surgical information.

It is a quick reference on a wide range of dermatologic diseases including concise clinical information on diagnostic features, lab findings and practical management as well as key surgical anatomy and pearls on lasers, basic science and pharmacology. Also included are notable dermatologic/dermpath mnemonics and a comprehensive quick reference of cutaneous disease and syndrome associations.

In all, this book provides a comprehensive collection of dermatology and dermatopathology signs and concise guidance on their significance, associated clinical and laboratory findings, as well as an extensive compilation of board review essentials.

EDITOR-IN-CHIEF
Joshua E. Lane, M.D., is Clinical Assistant Professor, Departments of Internal Medicine (Dermatology) and Surgery at Mercer University School of Medicine.

EDITORIAL BOARD
Jack L. Lesher, Jr., M.D., is Chief and Professor of the Division of Dermatology at the Medical College of Georgia.

Loretta S. Davis, M.D., is Professor of Dermatology at the Medical College of Georgia.

David E. Kent, M.D., is Clinical Assistant Professor of Medicine (Dermatology) at Mercer University School of Medicine.

David J. Cohen, M.D., is Chief of the Division of Dermatology at Mercer University School of Medicine.

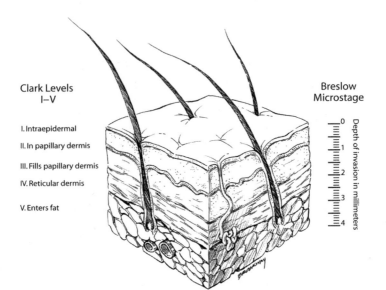

Clark Levels I–V

I. Intraepidermal

II. In papillary dermis

III. Fills papillary dermis

IV. Reticular dermis

V. Enters fat

Breslow Microstage

Depth of invasion in millimeters

0

1

2

3

4

Pocket Guide for Cutaneous Medicine and Surgery

JOSHUA E. LANE, M.D.
Clinical Assistant Professor
Departments of Internal Medicine (Dermatology) and Surgery
Mercer University School of Medicine

Clinical Instructor
Division of Dermatology
The Medical College of Georgia

EDITORIAL BOARD

JACK L. LESHER, JR., M.D.
Professor and Chief
Division of Dermatology
The Medical College of Georgia

LORETTA S. DAVIS, M.D.
Professor, Division of Dermatology
The Medical College of Georgia

DAVID E. KENT, M.D.
Mercer University School of Medicine
The Medical College of Georgia

Clinical Instructor
Division of Dermatology
The Medical College of Georgia

DAVID J. COHEN, M.D.
Clinical Assistant Professor and Chief
Department of Internal Medicine (Dermatology)
Mercer University School of Medicine

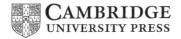

CAMBRIDGE
UNIVERSITY PRESS

CAMBRIDGE UNIVERSITY PRESS
Cambridge, New York, Melbourne, Madrid, Cape Town, Singapore, São Paulo

Cambridge University Press
40 West 20th Street, New York, NY 10011-4211, USA

www.cambridge.org
Information on this title: www.cambridge.org/9780521618137

First published 2006

Printed in the United States of America

A catalog record for this publication is available from the British Library.

Library of Congress Cataloging in Publication Data

Pocket guide for cutaneous medicine and surgery / Joshua E. Lane . . . [et al.].
    p. ; cm.
Includes bibliographical references and index.
ISBN-13: 978-0-521-61813-7 (pbk.)
ISBN-10: 0-521-61813-4 (pbk.)
1. Dermatology – Handbooks, manuals, etc.   2. Skin – Surgery –
Handbooks, manuals, etc.   I. Lane, Joshua E., 1972–   .
[DNLM: 1. Skin Diseases – Handbooks.   2. Skin Diseases – surgery – Handbooks.
WR 39 H2356   2006]
RL74.H36   2006
616.5 – dc22   2005024105

ISBN-13   978-0-521-61813-7 paperback
ISBN-10   0-521-61813-4 paperback

"Choose a job that you love and you'll never work a day in your life."   – Confucius

"If your ship doesn't come in, swim out to it."
                                    – Jonathan Winters

"There are three types of people: those who make things happen, those who watch things happen, and those who wonder what happened."   – Anonymous

"Whether you think you can or think you can't, you're right."
                                    – Henry Ford

"Be careful about reading health books. You might die of a misprint."   – Mark Twain

"The art of medicine consists in amusing the patient while nature cures the disease."   – Voltaire

"Surround yourself with the best people you can find, delegate authority, and don't interfere."   – President Ronald Reagan

CONTENTS

CONTRIBUTORS

Joshua E. Lane, M.D.
Clinical Assistant Professor
Departments of Internal Medicine (Dermatology) and Surgery
Mercer University School of Medicine
Macon, Georgia

Clinical Instructor
Division of Dermatology, Department of Medicine
The Medical College of Georgia
Augusta, Georgia

Jack L. Lesher, Jr., M.D.
Professor and Chief
Division of Dermatology, Department of Medicine
The Medical College of Georgia
Augusta, Georgia

Loretta S. Davis, M.D.
Professor
Division of Dermatology, Department of Medicine
The Medical College of Georgia
Augusta, Georgia

David E. Kent, M.D.
Clinical Assistant Professor
Department of Internal Medicine (Dermatology)
Mercer University School of Medicine
Macon, Georgia

Clinical Instructor
Division of Dermatology, Department of Medicine
The Medical College of Georgia
Augusta, Georgia

David J. Cohen, M.D.
Clinical Assistant Professor and Chief of Dermatology
Department of Internal Medicine (Dermatology)
Mercer University School of Medicine
Macon, Georgia

CLINICAL CONTRIBUTORS

I would like to dedicate this book to my wife and family for their continued encouragement and support and also to Dr. Kenneth Gresen, a compassionate mentor who showed me the beauty of medicine but left us too early.

I am grateful to the following colleagues and friends for their input and suggestions:

Tanda N. Lane, M.D.
Stephen E. Wolverton, M.D.
Richard Scher, M.D.
Anna N. Walker, M.D.
Jeffrey L. Stephens, M.D.
Christopher Peterson, M.D.
Christopher Kruse, M.D.
Cheryl Barnes, M.D.
John S. Pujals, M.D.
Daniel J. Sheehan, M.D.

Special thanks to Brian C. Brockway, M.S., Chief medical illustrator (Brockway Biomedical Studios [www.brockwaybiomedical.com]), for all medical illustrations. I also thank Leanne Powell for the scalp anatomy illustration.

I would also like to acknowledge Duane Whitaker, M.D., Alan R. Morgan, M.D., Jennifer G. Miller, M.D., Cheryl Jones, M.D., Kathy Lynn, M.D., Jacob Dudelzack, M.D., and Erik Hurst, M.D., for their assistance.

FOREWORD

The *Pocket Guide for Cutaneous Medicine and Surgery*, written by Joshua E. Lane, M.D., and collaborators from the Medical College of Georgia and Mercer University Schools of Medicine, is a wonderful addition to the dermatology literature. In addition to detailing all the knowledge required of a resident during that period, Dr. Lane took copious notes and gives countless pearls, factoids, and other useful information acquired during his dermatology residency. With guidance from his faculty at the Medical College of Georgia and his practice colleagues at Mercer University, he has created a compendium that should be invaluable to young dermatologists-in-training. There is also a great deal of information contained in this useful handbook that will be of value to practicing dermatologists as well as to trainees and practitioners in primary care disciplines. Dr. Lane has created a book that we had perhaps all wished that we had taken the time and made the effort to create for ourselves. I compliment Dr. Lane and his colleagues on this fine effort.

Joseph L. Jorizzo, MD

INTRODUCTION

The *Pocket Guide for Cutaneous Medicine and Surgery* is a book that I initially wrote for myself. It is a compilation of what I needed to know as a resident, a Fellow and a young attending, but perhaps could not remember without a little assistance. That was my impetus for writing this book.

Behind every author are a host of supportive mentors who dedicated their time and efforts to his or her education. This project is no exception. The efforts of my mentors from my undergraduate, graduate and postgraduate training are all reflected within this book. Doctors Carter, Gresen, Walker, Stephens, Lesher, Davis, Kent and Cohen guided me from each turning point of life to the next.

This handbook is designed for health care providers with a knowledge base of dermatology. It is meant to guide you while you interact with patients in the clinical setting, whether reminding you which labs to check for methotrexate or which never to avoid before your next surgery. That is why I wrote it and I hope that you find it equally as useful.

Joshua E. Lane, MD

Physical Examination

Admission Orders

A admit to . . . (floor, team, attending, intern)
D diagnosis
C condition
V vitals
A activity
A allergies
N nursing (strict I/O's, daily weights, chemstrips)
D diet (NPO / liquid / reg / cardiac / renal)
I intravenous fluids
S specific drugs
S symptomatic (DVT prophylaxis, Tylenol, Maalox, H_2-blocker)
E extra studies (EKG, CXR, consults)
L labs

Operative Note

Date of operation
Preop diagnosis (diagnosis and anatomic location)
Postop diagnosis
Operative procedure
Surgeons
Assistants
Anesthesia
Indications
Description of procedure
Findings

Specimens (orientation sutures)

EBL

Drains

Complications

Condition

Follow up and wound care instructions (activity, medications, diet)

Cranial Nerves

I olfactory
olfaction

II optic
vision, pupil light reflex

III oculomotor
innervates levator palpebra superioris

innervates 4 of 6 ocular muscles:
- superior rectus
- medial rectus
- inferior rectus
- inferior oblique

parasympathetic innervation of:
- ciliary muscle
- sphincter pupillae muscle

IV trochlear
innervates superior oblique muscle

V trigeminal

sensory innervation of face and scalp:

- opthalmic division
- maxillary division
- mandibular division

innervates muscles of mastication

tensors of tympanic membrane/palate

sensory for teeth, mucous membranes of mouth, nose, eye

VI abducens

innervates lateral rectus muscle

VII facial

all muscles of facial expression

innervates buccinator, platysma, stylohyoid, posterior belly of digastric, stapedius

parasympathetic innervation of salivary glands

sensory of concha of auricle

taste for anterior $\frac{2}{3}$ tongue

VIII vestibulocochlear

auditory and vestibular

IX glossopharyngeal

sensory innervation of:

- tympanic cavity
- eustachian tube
- tonsillar region of pharynx
- posterior $\frac{1}{3}$ of tongue (taste)

- external auditory canal and auricle

motor innervation of:

- stylopharyngeus muscle
- parotid (parasympathetic)

X vagal

pharyngeal muscles

- phonation
- swallow
- taste, elevates palate
- innervation of external auditory canal

XI spinal accessory

muscles of sternocleidomastoid, trapezius, muscles of soft
palate, pharynx, larynx

XII hypoglossal

extrinsic and intrinsic muscles of tongue

Dermatomes	
Clavicle	C4
Lateral upper arm	C5
Medial upper arm	T1,2
Thumb	C6
Middle and index fingers	C7
Third and fourth fingers	C8
Nipples	T4
Umbilicus	T10
Inguinal region	L1

Anterior and medial legs	L2–4
Foot	L4, L5, S1
Medial great toe	L5
Posterior and lateral legs	L5, S1, S2
Lateral foot and small toe	S1
Perineum	S2–4

Anterior and superior helix	Auriculotemporal nerve
Tragus	Auriculotemporal nerve
Occipital scalp	Greater occipital nerve
Posterior superior helix	Lesser occipital nerve
Posterior inferior helix	Greater auricular nerve
Posterior earlobe	Greater auricular nerve

Neurology

Function

C5	abduct arm
C6–8	adduct arm
C5,6	flex elbow
C7,8	extend elbow; flex/extend fingers
C6	pronate/supinate
C6,7	flex/extend wrist
T1	abduct/adduct fingers
L1–3	flex, adduct, medially rotate hip
L3,4	extend knee
L4,5	dorsiflex, invert ankle
L5, S1	evert ankle
S1	plantar flex

Oculomotor exam

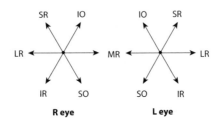

CN III	Superior division	SR	superior rectus
		LA	levator palpebrae superioris
	Inferior division	MR	medial rectus
		IO	inferior oblique
		IR	inferior rectus
CN IV		SO	superior oblique
CN VI		LR	lateral rectus

Anatomy

Anatomy – Trigeminal Nerve (CN V) – Facial Sensory

Ophthalmic nerve (CN V1)

Lacrimal	lateral upper eyelid, conjunctiva
Frontalis	
Supraorbital	anterior scalp, forehead, upper eyelids (pierces frontalis to reach skin)
Supratrochlear	medial upper eyelid, medial forehead, anterior scalp, nasal root, nasal bridge, upper nasal sidewalls (pierces corrugator to reach skin)
Nasociliary	
Infratrochlear	medial upper eyelid, nasal root, medial canthus, nasal bridge, upper nasal sidewalls
Anterior ethmoidal	
External nasal	branch of anterior ethmoidal supplies nasal dorsum, supratip, tip, columella
Posterior ethmoidal	

Maxillary nerve (CN V2)

Infraorbital	lower eyelid, nasal sidewall, nasal alae, upper lip, medial cheek, columella, anterior nasal mucous membrane (below infraorbital rim)
Zygomaticofacial	malar eminence
Zygomaticotemporal	preauricular cheek, anterior temple/scalp

Trigeminal Nerve (CN V)

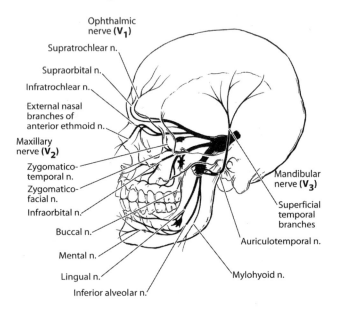

Ophthalmic nerve (**V₁**)
Supratrochlear n.
Supraorbital n.
Infratrochlear n.
External nasal branches of anterior ethmoid n.
Maxillary nerve (**V₂**)
Zygomatico-temporal n.
Zygomatico-facial n.
Infraorbital n.
Buccal n.
Mental n.
Lingual n.
Inferior alveolar n.
Mandibular nerve (**V₃**)
Superficial temporal branches
Auriculotemporal n.
Mylohyoid n.

Mandibular nerve (CN V3)

Auriculotemporal	anterior/superior ear (helix, tragus, temple, anterior half of external canal, tympanic membrane), temporoparietal scalp
Buccal	buccal mucosa/gingivum, cheek

Inferior alveolar

Mental   chin, lower lip, lower lip mucosa, nearby
                      gingiva (exits mental foramen ~2.5 cm
                      lateral to midline and inferior to 2nd
                      premolar)

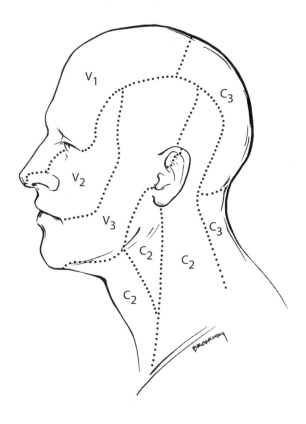

Anatomy – Facial Nerve (CN VII) – Facial Motor

Temporal
Innervates: frontalis, orbicularis oculi (with zygomatic branch), corrugator supercilii, temperoparietalis

Severed: ipsilateral brow ptosis and forehead paresis

Danger: as crosses mid-zygoma lateral to eyebrow

Zygomatic
Innervates: orbicularis oculi, procerus, nasalis, few mouth elevators

Severed: inability to close eyelids

Danger: buccal fat pad covered by SMAS and risorius

Buccal
Innervates: depressor septi; nasalis levator superioris alaeque nasi, levator labii superioris; buccinator, risorius, mouth elevators, zygomaticus major and minor; orbicularis oris, levator angulis oris

Severed: food remains in cheek

Danger: buccal fat pad

Mandibular
Innervates: risorius; orbicularis oris; depressor anguli oris; depressor labiii oris, levator anguli oris

Severed: drooping of ipsilateral lip and drooling

Danger: mandibular angle

Facial Nerve (CN VII)

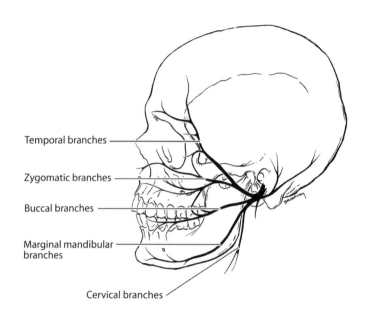

Temporal branches

Zygomatic branches

Buccal branches

Marginal mandibular branches

Cervical branches

Cervical

Innervates:	platysma and superior neck muscles
Severed:	decreased retraction of lower lip inferolaterally

CN VII:
- innervates all muscles of facial expression
- enters skull via stylomastoid foramen
- enters/traverses parotid gland

Anatomy – Arteries of the Face

External carotid artery (supplies majority of face and scalp)
Facial artery (chief artery of the face)
    Angular (supplies eyelids; joins ophthalmic artery)
    Lateral nasal
    Superior labial
    Inferior labial
Superficial temporal artery
    Frontal branch
    Parietal branch
    Zygomaticotemporal
    Middle temporal
    Transverse facial (anastomosis with branches of facial artery)
Occipital artery
Posterior auricular artery
Internal maxillary artery
    Infraorbital
    Buccal
    Mental

Internal carotid artery
Ophthalmic artery
    Supraorbital artery
    Supratrochlear artery
    Infratrochlear artery
    Dorsal nasal artery

Facial Arteries

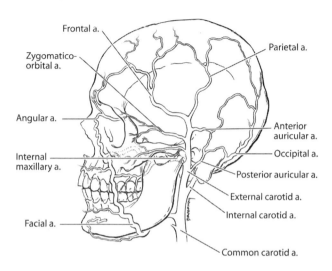

Frontal a.

Zygomatico-orbital a.

Parietal a.

Angular a.

Anterior auricular a.

Internal maxillary a.

Occipital a.

Posterior auricular a.

External carotid a.

Internal carotid a.

Facial a.

Common carotid a.

Anatomic Triangles of the Head and Neck

Anterior cervical triangle

Boundaries:	anterior median line of neck
	inferior border of mandible
	anterior border of sternocleidomastoid muscle
Veins:	internal jugular vein, retromandibular vein, facial vein, superior thyroid vein
Arteries:	superior thyroid artery, sternocleidomastoid branch of occipital artery, facial artery
Nerves:	greater auricular nerve, accessory nerve, facial nerve (cervical branch)
Muscles:	hyoid muscles:
	suprahyoid: mylohyoid, geniohyoid, stylohyoid, digastric
	infrahyoid: sternohyoid, sternothyroid, thyrohyoid, omohyoid)

Subdivisions of anterior cervical triangle:
Submental:
- bounded inferiorly by body of hyoid bone and laterally by anterior bellies of digastric muscles
- contains submental lymph nodes and anterior jugular vein

Submandibular:
- lies between inferior mandible and anterior/posterior portions of digastric muscle
- contains submandibular glands, submandibular lymph nodes, hypoglossal nerve (CN XII), parts of facial artery/vein

Neck Triangles

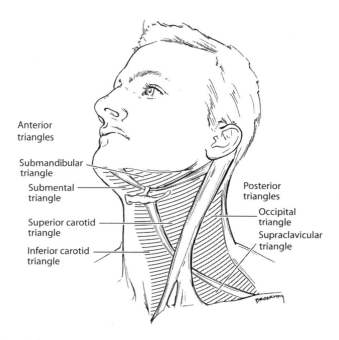

Anterior
triangles

Submandibular
triangle

Submental
triangle

Superior carotid
triangle

Inferior carotid
triangle

Posterior
triangles

Occipital
triangle

Supraclavicular
triangle

Carotid:

- bounded by superior belly of omohyoid, posterior belly of digastric and anterior border of sternocleidomastoid
- contains carotid artery, carotid sinus, carotid body, carotid sheath

Muscular:

- bounded by superior belly of omohyoid, anterior border of sternocleidomastoid and median plane of neck
- contains infrahyoid muscles, thyroid, parathyroid
- contains submental lymph nodes, anterior jugular vein

Posterior cervical triangle

Boundaries: posterior border of sternocleidomastoid
                  anterior border of trapezius
                  middle $\frac{1}{3}$ of clavicle
Veins: external jugular vein, subclavian vein
Arteries: subclavian artery, suprascapular artery, occipital
                  artery
Nerves: spinal accessory nerve, lesser occipital nerve,
                  supraclavicular brachial plexus, greater
                  auricular nerve
Muscles: splenius capitus, levator scapulae, scalenus
                  medius, scalenus posterior

Subdivisions of posterior cervical triangle:

Occipital triangle: contains occipital artery in apex and
   accessory nerve
Supraclavicular (subclavian) triangle: external jugular vein and
   suprascapular artery located superficially, subclavian artery
   located deep

Moore KL. *Clinically oriented anatomy, 3rd ed.* 1992, Williams and Wilkins, Philadelphia, pp. 783–852.

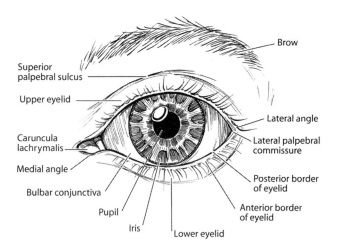

Brow

Superior
palpebral sulcus

Upper eyelid

Lateral angle

Caruncula
lachrymalis

Lateral palpebral
commissure

Medial angle

Posterior border
of eyelid

Bulbar conjunctiva

Anterior border
of eyelid

Pupil

Iris

Lower eyelid

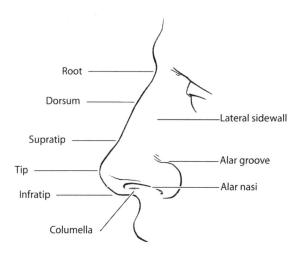

Root

Dorsum

Lateral sidewall

Supratip

Tip

Alar groove

Infratip

Alar nasi

Columella

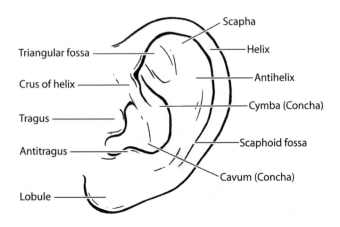

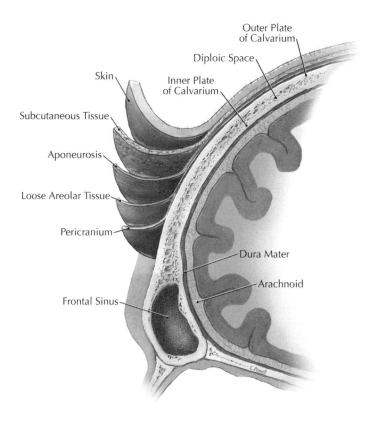

Dermatologic Surgery

Sutures

Absorbable:	Absorption (days)
Surgical gut (fast-absorbing)	21–42
Surgical gut (plain)	70
Surgical gut (chromic)	70–90
Polyglytone 6211 (Caprosyn: Syneture)	56
Polyglactin-910 (Vicryl: Ethicon) (Vicryl Rapide: Ethicon)	56–70
Lactomer (Polysorb: Syneture)	56–70
Polyglycolic acid (Dexon S/II: Syneture)	60–90
Glycomer 631 (Biosyn: Syneture)	90–110
Poliglecaprone 25 (Monocryl: Ethicon)	90–120
Polydioxanone (PDS II: Ethicon)	180
Polyglyconate (Maxon: Syneture)	180

Non-absorbable:

Silk (Perma-Hand: Ethicon; Sofsilk: Syneture)

Nylon (monofilament) (Ethilon: Ethicon; Monosof: Syneture)

Nylon (braided) (Nurulon: Ethicon; Surgilon: Syneture)

Polybutester (Novafil: Syneture)

Polypropylene (Prolene: Ethicon; Surgipro: Syneture)

Polyester (braided) (Mersilene: Ethicon; Dacron: Syneture)

(Teflon coated) (Ethibond: Ethicon; Ticron: Syneture)

Polyhexafluoropropylene-VDF (Pronova: Ethicon)

Weitzul S, Taylor RS. Suturing technique and other closure materials. In: Robinson JK, Hanke CW, Sengelmann RD, Siegel DM., eds. Surgery of the Skin. Philadelphia, Elsevier. 2005: pp. 227–230.

Needles

Needle	Curvature	Length	Syneture	Ethicon
CC[1]	$^3/_8$	11 mm	PC-13	P-1
		13 mm	PC-10*	PC-1*
		16 mm	PC-11*	PC-3*
		19 mm	PC-12	PC-5
RC[2]	$^3/_8$	11 mm	P-10	P-1
		13 mm	P-13	P-3
		16 mm	P-11	PS-3
		19 mm	P-12*	PS-2*
		24 mm	P-14	PS-1
	$^1/_2$	9 mm	P-21	P-2***
		13 mm	P-22	PS-5
RC[2]	$^1/_2$	15 mm	P-24	PS-4
		19 mm	C-13**	FS-2**
		24 mm	C-14	FS-1

[1] *CC = conventional cutting needle* (▲)
[2] *RC = reverse cutting needle* (▼)

* *Representative facial cosmetic needles*
** *Representative biopsy needle*
*** *Useful for vessel ligature in small anatomic locales (periorbital)*

Weitzul S, Taylor RS. Suturing technique and other closure materials. In: Robinson JK, Hanke CW, Sengelmann RD, Siegel DM., eds. Surgery of the Skin. Philadelphia: Elsevier. 2005: pp. 230–232.

Electrosurgery

Electrocautery   Not true electrosurgery
                             Heated filament transfers heat
                             No electric current transferred to patient
                             Useful with implantable cardiac devices

Monoterminal (1 contact between device & patient):

Electrodessication   Electrode contacts tissue
                             Low amperage / high voltage
                             Dampened wave form

Electrofulguration   Electrode above tissue (spark)
                             Low amperage / high voltage
                             Dampened wave form

Biterminal (2 contacts between device & patient):

Electrocoagulation   Thermal coagulation
                             High amperage / low voltage
                             Dampened waveform

Electrosection   Cuts through tissue
                             High amperage / low voltage
                             Undamped sinusoidal waveform

Soon S and Washington CV. Electrosurgery, electrocoagulation, electrofulguration, electrodessication, electrosection, electrocautery. In: Robinson JK, Hanke CW, Sengelmann RD, Siegel DM., eds. Surgery of the Skin. Philadelphia: Elsevier. 2005: p. 182.

Antiseptic Cleansers

Chlorhexidine (Hibiclens^{TM})
- disrupts cell membranes
- excellent gram-positive and good gram-negative coverage
- intermediate onset (~1 min. scrub)
- ototoxicity and keratitis
- residual chemical activity on skin
- antimicrobial activity not affected by blood

Hexachlorophene (pHisoHex^{TM})
- good gram-positive coverage only
- can be absorbed through skin → neurotoxicity in infants

Iodine / Iodophores (Betadine)
- iodine + surfactant → iodophore
- oxidation/substitution by free iodide (active agent)
- excellent gram-positive and good gram-negative coverage
- intermediate onset
- inactivated by blood and serum products

Isopropyl alcohol (70%)
- denatures proteins
- good gram-positive/negative coverage (mainly gram-positive)
- most rapid onset
- caution with lasers (flammable)

Triclosan
- disrupts cell wall
- good gram-positive/negative coverage
- intermediate onset

Occlusive Wound Dressings

Hydrogel

Description: • composed of polymer/copolymer and ≤95% water

• donates moisture to dehydrated tissue

• absorbs some moisture of exudating wound

• 2 types: amorphous and sheet

• non-particulate; non-toxic; non-adherent

Indications: • rehydrating sloughy/necrotic tissue

• enhancing autolytic debridement

• marked cooling effect; partial thickness wounds

Application: apply cover with 2° dressing (foam, film)

Limitations: may macerate wounds with high exudate levels

Products: Solugel, Vigilon, Tegagel, Curagel, Clearsite

Hydrocolloid

Description: • suspension of gel-forming polymer

• gums and adhesives on film/foam backing

• promotes moist wound environment

• aid autolytic debridement

• no particulate/toxic components

• waterproof and resistant to bacteria

• impermeable to oxygen

Indications: lightly/moderately exudative wounds

Application: warm in hand prior to application to increase activity of adhesive; no 2° dressing needed; wear 3–7 days

Limitations: limited fluid handling capacity
Products: Duoderm, NuDerm, Comfeel

Foam

Description: • porous, single/multiple layered dressings
                   • high fluid handling capacity (less maceration)
                   • insulating and permeable to moisture vapor
                     and gases
                   • non-adherent; non-particulate; non-toxic
                   • highly conformable and provides
                     cushioning/protection
Indications: light to highly exudative wounds; 2° dressing
Application: applied as 1° or 2°; change 2–3 days
Limitations: non-adhesive; require 2° dressing; not waterproof
Products: Allevyn, Flexzan, Hydrasorb, Lyofoam Vigifoam

Film

Description: • thin (polyurethane) membrane (adhesive on
                     1 side)
                   • permeable to moisture vapor and gases
                   • waterproof; bacteriaproof; elastic, conformable
                   • adhesive sticks to skin but not moist wounds
Indications: 2° dressing over foams, hydrogels, alginates;
                     waterproof; prevention of pressure wounds
Application: may apply for up to 1 week
Limitations: not suitable for infected wounds or deep wounds
Products: Tegaderm, Bioclusive, Omniderm, Transeal

Alginates

Description: • fibrous products derived from seaweed
- composed of calcium and sodium salts of alginic acid
- calcium alginate (solid) transforms (ion exchange) to sodium alginate (soluble) → absorbs exudate to form non-adherant gel
- promotes moist wound environment
- calcium ions → platelet aggregation and coagulation

Indications: moderate to highly exudative wounds; heavy bleeding

Application: • cover with 2° dressing
- may require sterile saline for removal
- may use on infected wounds

Limitations: • only for moderate to highly exudative wounds
- may dehydrate wounds with lower exudate levels
- D/C if dressing does not gel completely
- some may have tendency to wick laterally

Products: Algiderm, Algisite, Algisorb, Kaltostat, Seasorb, Sorbsan

Hydroactive

Description: • like hydrocolloid but traps fluid within matrix and swells
- adhesive matrix secured by film dressing
- non-adherant; waterproof; resistant to bacteria

Indications: moderate to high level of exudate

Application: apply with 3–4 cm intact skin around wound

Limitations: not indicated for low-level exudate or clinical infection
Products: Cutinova, Biatain

Hydrofiber
Description:
- similar to alginates (but carboxymethyl cellulose)
- absorb large amounts of fluid and forms gel similar in appearance to sheet hydrogel
- less likely to dry out; non-particulate; not hemostatic

Indications: highly exudative wounds
Application: similar to alginates (no lateral wicking)
Limitations: only for highly exudative wounds
Products: Aquacel

Zinc paste bandages
Description:
- open weave bandage with zinc oxide paste
- zinc thought to stimulate epithelialization
- beneficial in treatment of venous eczema

Indications: used on chronic wounds and final stages of healing
Application: requires 2° dressing; may leave for up to 7 days
Limitations: messy; difficult to work with; may give green tinge to wound/dressing; may contain allergenic preservatives
Products: Steripaste, Viscopaste, Flexidress®, Gelocast

Skin Grafts

Terminology

imbibition: 24–48 hours; graft sustained by plasma exudate via passive diffusion of nutrients

inosculation: 48–72 hours; linkage of existing vessels

neovascularization: newly formed vessels enter from perimeter and wound bed

Types:

Split Thickness Skin Grafts (STSG)

- use dermatome to harvest graft:
  - **thin:** 0.125–0.275 mm (0.005–0.011 inches)
  - **medium:** 0.275–0.4 mm (0.012–0.016 inches)
  - **thick:** 0.4–0.75 mm (0.016–0.03 inches)
- good for large areas with marginal vascular supply
- acts as "biological band-aid"
- risk of wound contracture
- decreased risk of graft failure
- cosmetically inferior to FTSG

Full Thickness Skin Grafts (FTSG)

- harvest via excision
- requires adequate vascular supply
- little wound contracture
- cosmetically superior to STSG

Chemical Peels

Superficial (depth of papillary dermis)

    Alpha-hydroxy acids

    CO_2 slush

    Jessner's solution (salicylic acid, lactic acid, resorcinol)

    Trichloracetic acid 10–30%

    Resorcinol

    Salicylic acid

    Glycolic acid

    Tretinoin

Medium (depth of upper reticular dermis)

    Trichloroacetic acid 45%

    Solid CO_2 and Trichloroacetic acid 35%

    Monheit peel (Jessner's peel + TCA 35%)

    70% glycolic acid and Trichloroacetic acid 35%

    89% phenol solution (aqueous)

Deep (depth of midreticular dermis)

    Baker's formula (phenol, water, liquid soap, croton oil)

    Trichloroacetic acid >50%

    Phenol

Botox Cosmetic

- supplied in 100 U vials (contains 100 U *Clostridium botulinum* type A neurotoxin + 0.5 mg human albumin + 0.9 mg NaCl)
- reconstitute with sterile, non-preservative normal saline

Diluent added	Dose (U/0.1 ml)
1 ml	10 U
2 ml	5 U
3 ml	3.3 U
4 ml	2.5 U

- use within 4 hours (store at 2–8 °C)
- injections of 0.1 ml
- avoid injection near levator palpebrae superioris
- do not inject closer than 1 cm above central eyebrows
- BOTOX interferes with ACh release
- H chain binds neurotoxin selectively to cholinergic terminal
- L chain acts within cell to prevent ACh release
- toxin A → cleaves SNAP-25
- toxin B → cleaves VAMP (synaptobrevin)

Topical Anesthesia

Anesthetic	Components	Vehicle	Onset (min.)
EMLA	2.5% lidocaine	oil in water	60–120
	2.5% prilocaine		
LMX 4	4% lidocaine	liposomal	30–60
LMX 5	5% lidocaine	liposomal	30–60

Notes

- may achieve effective anesthesia with 25 min. application
- recommend 60 min. application under occlusive dressing
- depth of analgesia at 60 min. approximates 3 mm
- depth of analgesia at 120 min. approximates 5 mm
- risk of methemoglobinemia with prilocaine (caution in infants)
- risk of alkaline injury to cornea with EMLA

Soriano TT, Lask GP, Dinehart SM. Anesthesia and analgesia. In: Robinson JK, Hanke CW, Sengelmann RD, Siegel DM., eds. Surgery of the Skin. Philadelphia, Elsevier. 2005: pp. 44–45.

Local Anesthesia

		Onset (min.)	Duration (min.)	Max dose[1] (mg/kg)
Without epinephrine				
Amides	Bupivacaine	2–10	120–240	2.5
	Etidocaine	3–5	240–360	4.5
	Lidocaine	<1	30–120	5
	Mepivacaine	3–20	30–120	6
	Prilocaine	5–6	30–120	7
Esters	Procaine	5	15–30	10
	Tetracaine	7	120–240	2
With epinephrine[2,3]				
Amides	Bupivacaine	2–10	240–480	3
	Etidocaine	3–5	240–360	6.5
	Lidocaine	<1	60–400	7
	Mepivacaine	3–20	60–400	8
	Prilocaine	5–6	60–400	10
Esters	Procaine	5	30–90	14
	Tetracaine	7	240–480	2

[1] Based on 70 kg patient
[2] Full vasoconstriction with epinephrine requires 7–15 min.
[3] Epinephrine is category C

Leal-Khouri et al. Local and topical anesthesia. In: Nouri K, Leal-Khouri S., eds. Techniques in Dermatologic Surgery. New York: Mosby. 2003: p. 49.

Soriano TT, Lask GP, Dinehart SM. Anesthesia and analgesia. In: Robinson JK, Hanke CW, Sengelmann RD, Siegel DM., eds. Surgery in the Skin. Philadelphia: Elsevier. 2005: p. 41.

Local Anesthesia

Injectable Local Anesthetics
Lidocaine Maximum Dosing
With Epinephrine: 7.0 mg/kg
Without Epinephrine: 4.5 mg/kg
Tumescent: 55 mg/kg

(0.5%, 1%, 2% ± 1:100,000 or 1:200,000 epinephrine)
Buffered: 1 ml 8.4% $NaHCO_3$ + 10 ml anesthetic (↑ pH to 7.3)

Tumescent ingredients: lidocaine, bicarbonate, epinephrine

Bupivacaine Maximum Dosing
With Epinephrine: 225 mg
Without Epinephrine: 175 mg

(0.25% ± 1:200,000 epinephrine)

Dosing Calculation:
1% = 1 g/100 ml → 10 mg/cc
2% = 2 g/100 ml → 20 mg/cc

	Esters	**Amides**
Metabolism	plasma cholinesterase	hepatic dealkylation
Excretion	renal	renal
Allergy	infrequent (>amides)	rare
Anesthetics	Benzocaine	Bupivacaine
	Chlorprocaine	Dibucaine
	Cocaine	Etidocaine
	Procaine	Lidocaine
	Tetracaine	Mepivicaine
		Prilocaine

Contraindications:
- severe blood pressure instability
- h/o true anesthetic allergy
- psychologic instability
- renal (esters) or hepatic (amides) disease
- esters cross-react with PABA

Alternatives:
- substitute amide for ester
- Benadryl 12.5 mg/ml
- bacteriostatic saline

Notes: Prilocaine: risk of methemoglobinemia
Bupivacaine: risk of cardiotoxicity (>lidocaine)
Bupivacaine cannot be buffered (precipitation)

Brodland DG, Huether MJ. Local anesthetics. In: Wolverton SE, ed. Comprehensive Dermatologic Drug Therapy. Phildadelphia: W.B. Saunders, Co. 2001: 739.

Klein JA. Tumescent technique. Tumescent anesthesia and microcannular liposuction. Mosby, 2000.

Lidocaine Toxicity

- marked by high serum concentrations → CNS/CVS toxicity
- biphasic toxicity:
  - excitatory: tingling, numbness, altered mental status, seizures
  - depressive: cessation of convulsions, unconsciousness, respiratory depression/arrest
- high concentrations block cardiac Na^+ channels
  - lidocaine commonly associated with sinus tachycardia
  - bupivacaine may cause ventricular tachycardia and fibrillation
- signs of lidocaine toxicity:
  - first sign is drowsiness ± dysarthria, lightheadedness, vertigo, circumoral/tongue numbness
  - may progress to tinnitus, difficult focusing, agitation
  - dysgeusia, nausea, tachypnea, facial twitching
  - generalized tonic/clonic seizures
- serum concentration >6 µg/ml may cause CNS symptoms
- concurrent use of cytochrome P450 3A4 inhibitors can increase serum lidocaine levels (see p. 209)
- treatment → SAVED mneunomic:
  S → stop injection
  A → airway
  V → ventilate
  E → evaluate circulation
  D → drugs

Poterack KA. Lidocaine toxicity. 2002. Emedicine (www.emedicine.com)

Soriano TT, Lask GP, Dinehart SM. Anesthesia and analgesia. In: Robinson JK, Hanke CW, Sengelmann RD, Siegel DM., eds. Surgery of the Skin. Philadelphia: Elsevier. 2005: pp. 54–56.

Antibiotic Prophylaxis

Class	Description	Infection	Prophylaxis
I	Clean	<5%	No
II	Clean-contaminated	~10%	Yes
III	Contaminated	20–30%	Yes
IV	Infected	30–40%	Yes

Risk factors:

preoperative shaving   diabetes
long duration   malnutrition
anergy   immunosuppression
obesity   remote infections

Indications for antibiotic prophylaxis (AHA guidelines):

High risk

- History of prosthetic heart valve
- History of endocarditis or cyanotic congenital heart disease
- History of systemic pulmonary shunts (surgically implanted)

Moderate risk

- Patent ductus arteriosus
- Valvular dysfunction (rheumatic heart disease, mitral valve prolapse with regurgitation)
- Orthopedic prostheses
- Ventriculoatrial/peritoneal shunts
- NOT routinely recommended for incision or biopsy of surgically scrubbed non-infected skin

Antibiotic Prophylaxis

Indications:

1. Prevention of endocarditis or prosthesis infection
2. Prevention of surgical site infection

Antibiotics: (administer 30–60 min. before surgery):

Cephalexin	2 g
Dicloxacillin	2 g
Clindamycin	600 mg
Azithromycin	500 mg
Clarithromycin	500 mg
Amoxicillin	2 g (oral/nasal cases)

Maragh SL, Otley CC, Roenigk RK et al. Antibiotic prophylaxis in dermatologic surgery: updated guidelines. Dermatol Surg 2005; 31: 81–93.

Babcock MD and Grekin RC. Antibiotic use in dermatologic surgery. Dermatol Clin 2003; 21: 337–348.

Rabb DC, Lesher JL. Antibiotic prophylaxis in cutaneous surgery. Dermatol Surg 1995; 21: 550–554.

Hass AF and Grekin RC. Antibiotic prophylaxis in dermatologic surgery. J Am Acad Dermatol 1995; 32: 155–176.

ACC/AHA Guidelines for the Management of Patients with Valvular Heart Disease. ACC/AHA Task Force Report JACC 1998; 32: 1486–1588.

Nouri et al. Aseptic techniques. In: Nouri K, Leal-Khouri S., eds. Techniques in Dermatologic Surgery. New York: Mosby. 2003: pp. 43–46

Coagulation Cascade

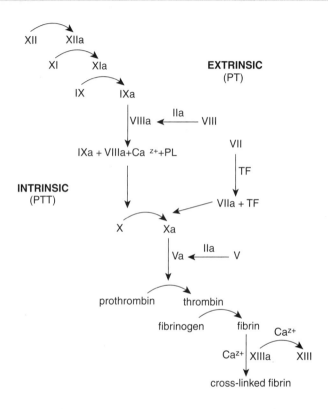

- intrinsic pathway factors XI and XII: necessary for *in vitro* coagulation but not critical for *in vivo* hemostasis
- factor XIII is not measured by most routine coagulation studies

Anticoagulants and Mechanisms

Aspirin:
- inhibits prostaglandin synthesis
- irreversibly inhibits platelet aggregation

Clopidogrel (Plavix):
- inhibits ADP binding to platelet receptors

Dalteparin (Fragmin):
- binds antithrombin III to accelerate activity
- inhibits thrombin and factor Xa

Dipyridamole (Persantine)
- inhibits platelet adhesion (mechanism unknown)

Enoxaparin (Lovenox)
- binds antithrombin III to accelerate activity
- inhibits thrombin and factor Xa

Heparin
- inhibits thrombin and factor Xa
- inhibits conversion of fibrinogen to fibrin

NSAIDs
- inhibit cyclooxygenase and lipoxygenase
- reduce prostaglandin synthesis

Ticlopidine (Ticlid)
- inhibits ADP-induced platelet-fibrinogen binding

Warfarin (Coumadin):
- inhibits vitamin K-dependent coagulation factors (II, VII, IX, X, proteins C, S)

Aggrenox (aspirin + extended release dipyridamole)

OTC anticoagulants: feverfew, garlic, gingko, ginseng, St. John's wort, vitamin E

Hemostasis and Diagnostics

Partial thromboplastin time (PTT; activated PTT; APTT)

Collection: blue stopper tube (3.2% sodium citrate)

Use: monitoring unfractionated heparin therapy, detecting coagulation inihibitors and deficiencies of intrinsic and common pathways

Reference: 25–34 s

Critical: ≥120 s

Therapeutic range: heparin (iv) 68–100 s; (sq) 52–75 s

Prothrombin time (PT/INR)

Collection: blue stopper tube (3.2% sodium citrate)

Use: monitoring oral anticoagulation therapy (Coumadin) and to detect deficiency of extrinsic and common pathways

Reference: 12.3 – 14.2 s / INR 1.0

Critical: >50 s

Therapeutic range: S/P venous thromboembolism, MI, Afib → INR 2–3

mechanical heart valve → INR 2.5–3.5

Anti-Xa (unfractionated heparin anti-Xa; LMWH anti-Xa)
Collection: blue stopper tube (3.2% sodium citrate)
Use: monitoring unfractionated heparin therapy and LMWH
Reference: 0.0 anti-Xa heparin units/ml plasma
Critical: _____
Therapeutic range: therapeutic → 0.3–0.7
prophylaxis → 0.1–0.4
LMWH (therapeutic) → 0.4–1.0
LMWH (prophylaxis) → 0.2–0.4

Closure time – PFA – 100 (platelet function assay)
Collection: blue stopper tube (3.2% buffered sodium citrate)
Use: monitoring bleeding time
measures qualitative and quantitative platelet
defects detects platelet dysfunction induced by:
- intrinsic platelet defects
- von Willebrand disease
- exposure to platelet inhibiting agents (aspirin)

Reference: screen (collagen/epinephrine [COL/EPI]) 75–160 s
(if abnormal, then collagen/ADP [COL/ADP] 55–100 s)

Notes: not designed to predict bleeding time during surgery
  abnormal results may occur in patients with anemia,
  thrombocytopenia, high fat diets, increased ESR

	COL/EPI	COL/ADP
Normal	normal	normal
Aspirin	abnormal	normal
Plavix	abnormal	abnormal
von Willebrand disease	abnormal	abnormal
Glanzmann's thrombasthenia	abnormal	abnormal

Bleeding Disorders

Plt	BT	PTT	PT	Diagnosis	Etiology
↓	↑	–	–	Thrombocytopenia	ITP Drugs
–	↑	↑	–	vW disease	–
–	↑	–	–	Qualitative platelet defect	Drugs Uremia Inherited
–	–	↑	–	Intrinsic defect	Hemophilia Factor VIII def vW disease Lupus anticoag
–	–	↑	↑	Common defect	Liver disease Vitamin K def DIC Heparin
–	–	–	↑	Extrinsic defect	Factor VII def Coumadin
–	–	–	–		Hereditary telangiectasia Allergic purpura

Legend:

Plt	platelet
BT	bleeding time (replaced by closure time [PFA-100])
PTT	prothrombin time
PT	protime

Lasers and Light

Lasers

Infrared	λ (nm)
CO_2 (targets H_2O)	10,600
Erbium:YAG	2,940
Neodynium:YAG	1,064
Diode	810

Visible

Red:	Q-switched alexandrite	755
	Q-switched ruby	694
Yellow:	Flashlamp pulsed yellow dye	585–600
	Copper vapor	578
	Krypton	520, 568
Green:	KTP (Potassium titanyl phosphate)	532
	Freq-doubled Nd:YAG (QS)	532
	Continuous wave Argon	488, 514, 630
	Flashlamp pumped green-dye	504
Blue:	Argon (continuous)	488

Ultraviolet

Pulsed Excimer	193, 308, 351

Terminology:

Energy	J
Dose	J/cm^2
Power	W (J/s)
Irradiance	W/cm^2

UV Spectrum Wavelengths

UV Spectrum	Wavelength
Radiowave	>1 mm
Microwave	1 mm – 25 µm
Infrared	>760 nm
Visible	400–760 nm
UVA 1 (long wave)	340–400 nm
UVA 2 (short wave)	320–340 nm
UVB	290–320 nm
UVC	200–290 nm
X-rays	1 nm – 1 pm
Gamma rays	<1 pm

narrow band UVB: 311 nm
pyrimidine dimer formation greatest at 290–310 nm

SPF	UVB blocked
2	50%
4	75%
8	87.5%
15	93.3%
20	95%
30	96.7%
45	97.8%
50	98%

Microbiology and Immunology

Bacteriology

Gram Positive

Cocci	*Streptococcus*	*Staphylococcus*
Rods (aerobe)	*Bacillus*	
Rods (anaerobe)	*Clostridium*	
Rods (non-spore)	*Corynebacterium*	*Listeria*
	Actinomyces	*Nocardia*

Gram Negative

Cocci	*Neisseria*	
Rods (respiratory)	*Haemophilus*	*Bordatella*
	Legionella	
Rods (zoonotic)	*Brucella*	*Francisella*
	Pasteurella	*Yersinia*
Rods (enteric)	*Escherichia*	*Enterobact*
	Serratia	*Klebsiella*
	Salmonella	*Shigella*
	Proteus	
Rods (curved)	*Pseudomonas*	*Vibrio*
Rods (anaerobe)	*Bacteriodes*	
Acid-fast	*Mycobacterium*	
	Nocardia	
Obligate intracellular	*Rickettsia*	*Chlamydia*
Spirochetes	*Treponema*	*Borrelia*
	Leptospira	
Wall-less	*Mycoplasma*	

Classification of Mycobacteria

Group I   photochromogens
            yellow pigment on Löwenstein-Jensen culture
            medium (with light exposure at 37° C)
            M. kansaii, M. marinum, M. simiae

Group II   scotochromogens
            yellow-orange pigment (even with culture in dark)
            M. scrofulaceum, M. szulgai, M. gordonae,
                M. xenopi

Group III   nonphotochromogens
            do not produce pigment
            M. avium-intracellulare complex, *M. haemophilum,*
                M. ulcerans, M. malmoense

Group IV   rapid growers
            do not produce identifying pigment
            rapid growth rate of 3–5 days
            M. fortuitum, M. chelonei, M. abscessus

Odom RB, James WD, Berger TG. Andrews' Diseases of the Skin, 9 ed.
Philadelphia: W.B. Saunders, Co. 2000: p. 426.

DNA Viruses

Virus	Disease	DNA	Envelope
Herpes-		ds	yes
Alpha			
Simplex	HSV-1 and 2		
Varicella	VZV (HSV-3)		
Beta			
CMV	CMV (HSV-5)		
Roseola	HSV-6		
Gamma			
Lympho	EBV (HSV-4)		
Hepadna-	HBV	ds	yes
Adeno-	pharyngitis, ARD	ds	no
Papo-			no
Papilloma-	papilloma	ds	
Polyoma-	BK, JC	ss	
Parvo-	B-19	ss	no
Pox-	molluscum, orf variola, vaccinia	ds	yes

RNA Viruses

Virus	Disease	RNA	Env
Toga-		ss	yes
Alpha-	E/W/V encephalitis		
Rubivi-	rubella virus (German measles)		
Corono-		ss	yes
Retro-	HIV, HTLV (+ sense)	ss	yes
Picorna-		ss	no
Entero-	polio, coxsackie		
Rhino-	rhinovirus		
Hepato-	HAV		
Calici-		ss	no
Flavi-	HCV, Jap/SL encephalitis	ss	yes
	Dengue, Yellow fever, W Nile		
Reo-		ds	no
Orthomyxo-	influenza virus	ss	yes
Paramyxo-		ss	yes
Paramyxo-	parainfluenza 1 and 3		
Rubula-	parainfluenza 2 and 4		
Morbilli-	measles		
Pneumo-	RSV		
Rhabdo-	rabies	ss	yes
Bunya-	CA encephalitis, Hantavirus	ss	yes
Arena-	LCM, Lassa virus	ss	yes
Filo-	Ebola-Marburg virus	ss	yes

HPV Types and Disease

Disease	HPV Types
Actinic keratosis	36
Bowen's disease	34
Bowenoid papulosis	16, 18, 33, 34, 42
Butcher's warts	7
Cervical cancer	16, 18, 31, 33, 35, 39
Condyloma acuminata	6, 11, 16, 18
Condyloma, flat	42
Epidermodysplasia verruciformis	5, 8–10, 12, 14, 15, 17, 19–29, 36, 47, 50
Genital papilloma	42
Giant condyloma acuminata of Buschke and Lowenstein	6, 11
Laryngeal papilloma	6, 11, 16, 18
Laryngeal carcinoma	6, 11, 30, 40
Keratoacanthoma	36, 37
Malignant melanoma	38
Oral focal epithelial hyperplasia (Heck's disease)	13, 32
Stucco keratoses	9, 16, 23b
Verrucous carcinoma of the foot	2
Verruca, filiform	2
Verruca, mosaic (plantar)	2 (4, 60, 63, 65)
Verruca, palatal	2
Verruca, plana	3, 10, 28, 41, 49
Verruca, plantar/palmar/myrmecia	1
Verruca, vulgaris	2, 7

Smallpox

Caused by variola (poxvirus)

Major Criteria:

- Febrile prodrome 1–4 days before rash: fever $\geq 101°F$ and at least one of following: prostration, headache, backache, chills, vomiting, severe abdominal pain, prodromal eruption in "swimming trunk" distribution
- Classic lesions: deep-seated, firm/hard, round well-circumscribed, vesicles/pustules (may become umbilicated/confluent)
- Lesions in same stage of development (unlike chickenpox)

Minor Criteria:

- Centrifugal distribution
- First lesions on oral mucosa/palate, face, forearms
- Appears toxic/moribund
- Slow evolution
- Lesions on palms/soles

Vaccination Timeline

Day	Cutaneous finding
3–4	Papule
5–6	Vesicle with surrounding erythema → vesicle with center
8–9	Well-formed pustule
12+	Pustule crusts over → scab
17–21	Scab detaches → scar

Complications of smallpox vaccination

- eczema vaccinatum (seen with eczematous patients)
- generalized vaccinia (children with IgM deficiency prone)
- vaccinia necrosum (usually infants <6 mo with immune deficiency)
- roseola vaccinia (symmetrical eruption macules, papules)
- congenital vaccinia (following vaccination in pregnancy)

Candida Antigen Therapy for Verrucae

- 0.1 ml *Candida* test Ag intradermal
- assess reaction at 48 hour (positive >5 mm)
- *Candida* antisera for injection (based on initial reaction):

induration (mm)	injection (ml)
5–20	0.3
21–40	0.2
>40	0.1

Exclusion criteria:
- prior allergy to *Candida* antisera
- pregnancy
- HIV type I
- iatrogenic immunosuppression
- primary immunosuppression
- generalized dermatitis

Notes:
- treat largest of multiple verrucae
- maximum of 3 treatments
- non-responders S/P 3 treatments → cryotherapy

Johnson SM et al. Intralesional injection of mumps or Candida skin test antigens: a novel immunotherapy for warts. *Arch Dermatol* 2001; 137: 451–455.

Squaric Acid Sensitization Therapy

- sensitize with 1–2% squaric acid dibutylester under occlusion to ~2 cm^2 area of normal skin on upper arm overnight
- patient may wash after 24 hour period
- may re-sensitize in 7–10 days if needed
- apply squaric acid to verruca after sensitized q 2 weeks

Exclusion criteria:

- intolerance to squaric acid
- pregnancy
- chronic allergic contact dermatitis
- systemic immunosuppression

Silverberg NB, Lim JK, Paller AS, Mancini AJ. Squaric acid immunotherapy for warts in children. *J Am Acad Dermatol* 2000; 42: 803–808.

Lee AN, Mallory SB. Contact immunotherapy with squaric acid dibutylester for the treatment of recalcitrant warts. *J Am Acad Dermatol* 1999; 41: 595–599.

Immunology

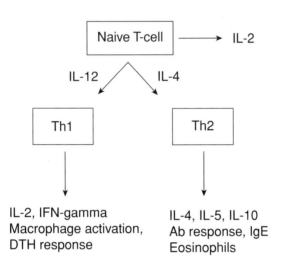

Examples:

Tuberculoid leprosy	Lepromatous leprosy
Cutaneous T-cell lymphoma	Sézary syndrome
Psoriasis	Atopic dermatitis

Note: Diseases classified as either Th1 or Th2 often have some components of both but can be classified based on the predominant cytokine profiles

Complement System

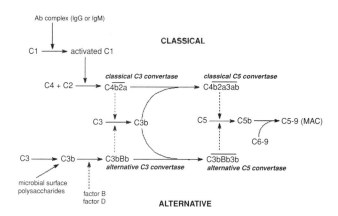

- classical pathway:
  - activated by IgG or IgM (Ag bound, not soluble)
  - IgM > IgG3 > IgG1 = IgG2 (IgG4 does not bind C1q)
- alternative pathway: activated without Ab
- MB lectin pathway: (structural similarity to C1q)
  - binds various pathogens: *Candida, Listeria, Neisseria, Cryptococcus, Salmonella*
- functions of complement proteins:
  - cell lysis: C5-C9
  - opsonization/phagocytosis: C3bi
  - vascular response: C5a > C3a > C4a
  - PMN activation: C5a
  - immune complex removal: classical pathway, C3b
  - B cell activation: C3bi

Deficiencies of early complement associated with autoimmune disease; late components associated with infection.

Clinical Pearls

Angioedema

	C1 INH Quantitative	C1 INH Qualitative	CH50	C1	C4	C2	C3
HAE type 1	↓↓	↓↓	nl/↓	nl	↓↓	↓	nl
HAE type 2	nl / ↑	↓↓	nl/↓	nl	↓↓	↓	nl
AAE type 1	↓↓	↓↓		↓	↓↓		
AAE type 2	nl / ↓	↓↓	↓↓	↓↓	↓↓	↓↓	nl

Legend: HAE (hereditary angioedema); AAE (acquired angioedema)

- subcutaneous edema, upper respiratory/GI tract involvement
- no pruritus and no urticaria
- screening test of choice is C4 (↓from continuous consumption)
- HAE type 1 – AD inheritance; ↓ production of normal C1-INH
- AAE type 1 associated with lymphoproliferative diseases
- AAE type 1 2° anti-idiotypic Ab to monoclonal Ig synthesized by B lymphocytes; treat with attentuated androgens

- AAE type 2 2° IgG$_1$ autoantibodies that bind to and interfere with function of C1-INH; treat with glucocorticoids

Gigli I and Rosen FS. Angioedema associated with Complement Abnormalities. In: Freedberg IM et al., eds. Fitzpatrick's Dermatology in General Medicine, 6 ed. New York, NY: McGraw-Hill. 2003:1139–1143.

Odom RB, James WD, Berger TG. Andrews' Diseases of the Skin, 9th ed., Philadelphia: W.B. Saunders, Co. 2000: p. 166.

Terminology of Skin Lesions

Primary Skin Lesions

Macule	small, flat discoloration
Papule	small (<1 cm)circumscribed, solid elevation
Nodule	large (1–2 cm)circumscribed, elevation
Tumor	large nodule (>2 cm)
Plaque	large (>1 cm) flat-topped elevation, often formed by confluence of papules
Pustule	small circumscribed elevation containing purulent material
Vesicle	small (<5 mm) collection of clear fluid
Bulla	large (>5 mm) collection of clear fluid
Telangiectasis	dilated superficial blood vessel
Wheal	irregular edematous plaque
Patch	macule with texture change

Secondary Skin Lesions

Scale	residual epidermal cells
Crust	scab
Erosion	focal loss of epidermis
Ulcer	focal loss of epidermis and dermis
Fissure	linear ulcer/erosion
Excoriation	traumatized area (often linear) (2° scratching)
Lichenification	thickening with accentuation of skin lines (2° rubbing)

Nail Terminology

Onycholysis	separation of distal nail plate from nail bed
Onychomadesis	separation of entire nail plate beginning proximally
Onychogryphosis	overgrowth of nail ("ram's horn" appearance)
Onychocryptosis	ingrown nail
Onychauxis	thick nail
Onychoschizia	splitting of nails into layers parallel to surface
Onychorrhexis	longitudinal ridging of nails
Onychomalacia	softening of nails
Brachyonychia	short, wide nails ("raquet nails" in Rubenstein-Taybi)
Koilonychia	spoon nails (iron deficiency; Plummer-Vinson; hyperthyroidism; hemochromotosis)
Platonychia	flattened nails
Hapalonychia	thinning of nail plate
Trachyonychia	rough nails
Beau's lines	horizontal ridges in nail plate (slow matrix proliferation during acute illness)
Mee's lines	associated with heavy metals and some chemotherapy
Half and Half nails	(Lindsay's nails) transverse white lines associated with renal disease (transverse white line in nail bed)

Terry's nails   transverse lines associated with liver
                        disease (whitening of nail bed)
Muehrckes' nails   pale bands on nailbed associated with
                        hypoalbuminemia
"Shoreline" nails   drug-induced exfoliative dermatitis
                        (alternating bands of nail plate
                        discontinuity and leukonychia)
Bilobed nails   only few reported cases
Yellow nails: yellow nail syndrome, *Candida*,
                        carotenemia, MTX, AZT
Blue nails: Wilson's disease, argyria, AZT, HIV,
                        antimalarials, busulfan
Red lunulae: carbon monoxide, CV disease, lupus,
                        alopecia areata

Nail pitting: psoriasis vulgaris, alopecia areata
Psoriasis: nail pitting, oil spots, onycholysis

Pediatric Dermatology

Rubeola (Measles)
- paramyxovirus
- 8–12 days post-exposure (no signs)
- prodrome: malaise, fever, cough, coryza, conjunctivitis; Koplik spots in 2–3 days after onset of symptoms
- erythematous maculopapular rash ~5 days after onset of symptoms (cephalocaudal progression)
- atypical measles (individual vaccinated with killed vaccine)

Rubella (German measles)
- rubella virus (RNA togavirus)
- no prodrome during incubation (14–21 days)
- erythematous, maculopapular, discrete rash (starts on face and spreads to body over 24°; resolves by day 3)
- lymphadenopathy (posterior cervical and suboccipital)
- ocular pain with upward and lateral gaze characteristic
- fever may accompany onset of erythema
- Forscheimer's spots – pinpoint rose-colored macules/petechia on soft palate

Roseola
- HHV 6 (>HHV7)
- abrupt fever days 3–5 (appears well)
- maculopapular rash on 3rd day (centrifugal) as fever deferresces; leukocytosis
- rash evolves in 12° and lasts 1–2 days
- 95% are 6 months to 2 years of age
- Berliner's sign – palpebral edema
- spread via oropharyngeal secretion

Erythema infectiosum (Fifth's disease)
- parvovirus B-19 (ssDNA)
- prodrome consists of fever, HA, pharyngitis, malaise
- slapped cheek appearance
- erythematous, reticulated, pruritic, macular rash (arms → trunk, legs) (reticulated hyperpigmentation)
- aplastic crisis in patients with hemoglobinopathies
- acute arthropathy in adults (and papular gloves and stockings)
- risk of hydrops fetalis and spontaneous abortion

Hand-foot-mouth disease
- coxsackie A16 virus; enterovirus 71
- prodrome of fever, anorexia, oral pain followed by oral mucosal ulcers and erythematous patches and vesicles on hands, feet, and buttocks

Varicella Zoster Virus (VZV)
- incubation: 10–21 days
- absent or mild prodrome
- vesicles in varying stages of development (cephalocaudal)
- immunocompromised children with VZV are given VZIG within 96° of exposure
- acyclovir reserved for immunocompromised with disseminated varicella
- contagious from 24° before onset of rash until all lesions are crusted over

Kawasaki disease (Mucocutaneous lymph node syndrome)

- systemic vasculitis of unknown etiology
- characteristic features:
    - fever of unknown origin for >5 days
    - acral/perineal erythema/desquamation
    - cervical nonsuppurative lymphadenopathy
    - edema/desquamation of hands and feet
    - conjunctivitis
    - strawberry tongue
- 3 phases:
    - acute: lasts 1–2 weeks
    - subacute: begins when fever, rash, LAD resolve; marked by desquamation and thrombocytosis; risk of arthritis, coronary aneurysms
    - convalescent: 6–8 weeks after onset; ESR normal
- treat with aspirin and IVIG

Scarlet fever

- usually associated with streptococcal pharyngitis
- erythrogenic toxins B and C most commonly seen
- highest incidence in children 2–10 (can occur in adults)
- fever, malaise, pharyngitis → exanthem 48° later (neck spreading down) → pinpoint papules (sandpaper feel; often spares palms and soles); circumoral pallor; accentutation in skin folds (Pastia's lines) → lasts ~5 days → desquamates (often in sheets)
- enanthem: pharyngitis, palatal petechia, white strawberry tongue → red strawberry tongue

Varicella Zoster Virus and Pregnancy

- maternal VZV infection within first 20 weeks gestation may result in congenital varicella syndrome
- VZIG should not be given once mother has developed varicella
- VZIG should be given for significant exposures within first 72–96 hours (use limited to seronegative women)
- if mother develops varicella 5 days before or 2 days after delivery → administration of VZIG is warrranted (consider iv acyclovir therapy)

Diagnosis of Systemic Lupus Erythematosus

Requires 4 of 11 for diagnosis:
Malar erythema (tends to spare nasolabial folds)

Discoid lupus erythematosus
Photosensitivity (patient history or examination)
Oral ulcers (oral/nasopharyngeal ulceration; usually painless)
Arthritis (nonerosive) involving ≥2 peripheral joints
   (characterized by tenderness, swelling or effusion)
Serositis (pericarditis or pleuritis)

Nephropathy
   persistent proteinuria >0.5 g/d or 3+ (or)
   cellular casts (red cell, hemoglobin, granular, tubular, mixed)
Neurologic disorder(seizures/psychosis in absence of drugs or
   metabolic derangements)

Hematologic disorder
   • hemolytic anemia with reticulocytosis or
   • leukopenia <4000/mm^3 on 2 occasions or
   • lymphopenia <1500/mm^3 on 2 occasions or
   • thrombocytopenia <100,000/mm^3

Immunologic disorder (+LE-prep; anti-DNA Ab or Sm Ag or
   false + for syphilis known to be + for ≥6 months)

Antinuclear antibody

Tan EM, Cohen AS, Fries JF, Masi AT, McShane DJ, Rothfield NF et al. The 1982 revised criteria for the classification of systemic lupus erythematosus. *Arthritis and Rheumatism* 1982; 25:1271–1277.

Useful Laboratory Tests in Evaluation of SLE

Complete blood count anemia, leukopenia, thrombocytopenia
Differential check for lymphopenia
ESR usually elevated (but nonspecific)
Creatinine $\pm$ elevated with renal involvement
Urinalysis check for proteinuria, hematuria, casts
RPR/VDRL false-positive test may occur with SLE

ANA 95% with SLE (use Hep-2 cell line)
dsDNA increased risk of renal disease
ssDNA sensitive but not specific
Sm highest specificity for SLE
nRNP decreased risk of renal disease
C3/C4 decreased with active disease
antiphospholipid Ab may occur with SLE
anti-histone Ab drug-induced lupus

Koopman WJ, Boulware DW, Heudebert GR. Clinical Primer of Rheumatology. Philadelphia: Lippincott Williams and Wilkins. 2003: p. 167.

Antinuclear antibodies

Pattern	Target	Antibody	Disorder
Homogeneous	Chromatin	anti-dsDNA	SLE
		anti-dsDNA	Drug-induced LE
		anti-histone	
Peripheral	Chromatin	anti-DNA	SLE
	Nuclear mem	anti-laminin	
Speckled/ fine	Nuclear RNP	anti-Sm	SLE (nephritis)
		anti-Ro/SSA	SCLE,Sjögren's
		anti-La/SSB	Sjögren's
		anti-U1RNP	SLE, MCTD
	Chromatin	anti-Ku	SLE, scleroderma
		anti-SCl-70	Scleroderma
Speckle/discrete	Chromatin	anti-centromere	CREST
Nucleolar	Nuclear RNP	anti-U3RNP	Scleroderma
	Nucleolar comp	anti-RNA Pol I	
		anti-Pm-SCl	

Jaworsky C. Connective tissue diseases. In: Elder D et al. Lever's Histopathology of the Skin. Philadelphia: Lippincott-Raven. 1997: p. 267.

Porphyrias

PORPHYRIAS

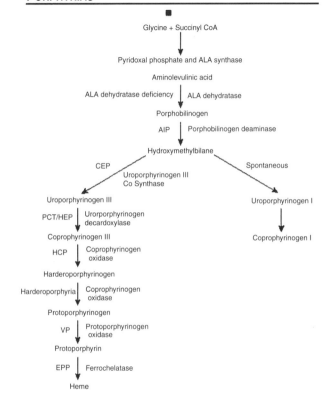

■

Glycine + Succinyl CoA

↓

Pyridoxal phosphate and ALA synthase

Aminolevulinic acid

ALA dehydratase deficiency │ ALA dehydratase

Porphobilinogen

AIP │ Porphobilinogen deaminase

↓

Hydroxymethylbilane

CEP ╱ Uroporphyrinogen III   Spontaneous ╲
Co Synthase

Uroporphyrinogen III   Uroporphyrinogen I

PCT/HEP │ Urorporphyrinogen   │
decardoxylase

Coprophyrinogen III   Coprophyrinogen I

HCP │ Coprophyrinogen
oxidase

Harderoporphyrinogen

Harderoporphyria │ Coprophyrinogen
oxidase

Protoporphyrinogen

VP │ Protoporphyrinogen
oxidase

Protoporphyrin

EPP │ Ferrochelatase

Heme

Porphyria Laboratory Evaluation

	EP[1]	EPP[2]	EC[3]	AIP[4]	PCT[5]	VP[6]	HC[7]	HEP[8]
Inher	AR	AD	AD	AD	AD	AD	AD	AR
Age	Child	Child	Child	Adult	Adult	Adult	Adult	Child
Cutan Immed	3+	2+	2+	−	−	−	−	2+
Cutan Delay	3+	−	−	−	2+	2+	1+	2+
Neuro	−	−	−	3+	−	2+	3+	−
RBC	URO COP	PROT	COP					PROT
Stool	COP	PROT	COP		COP PROT	PROT	COP	ISO
Urine	URO		COP	URO	ALA PBG	COP ALA, PBG	COP ALA PBG	URO ISO

[1] EP: erythropoietic porphyria – uroporphyrinogen III cosynthase
[2] EPP: erythropoietic protoporphyria – ferrochelatase
[3] Erythropoietic coproporphyria – coproporphyrinogen oxidase
[4] Acute intermittent porphyria – porphobilinogen oxidase
[5] Porphyria cutanea tarda – uroporphyrinogen decarboxylase
[6] Variegate porphyria – protoporphyrinogen oxidase
[7] Hereditary coproporphyria – coproporphyrinogen oxidase
[8] Hepatoerythropoietic porphyria – uroporphyrinogen decarbox

Mitochondrial: ALA synthase, Coprogen oxidase, Protogen oxidase, Ferrochelatase

Cytoplasmic: ALA dehydratase, Porphobilinogen deaminase, Urogen III synthase, Urogen decarboxylase

Bickers DR, Frank J. The Porphyrias. In: Freedberg IM et al., eds. Fitzpatrick's Dermatology in General Medicine, 6 ed. New York, NY: McGraw-Hill. 2003: p. 1437.

Epidermolysis Bullosa

Intraepidermal (*keratins 5 and 14 for most*)
   EB simplex, generalized (Koebner)
   EB simplex, localized (Weber-Cockayne)
   EB herpetiformis (Dowling-Meara)
   EB simplex (Ogna) (plectin)
   EB simplex with mottled pigmentation
   EB with muscular dystrophy (plectin; hemidesmosome)

Junctional (*intralamina lucida*) (laminin V)
   JEB atrophicans generalisata gravis (Herlitz; EB letalis)
   JEB atrophicans generalisata mitis
   JEB atrophicans localisata
   JEB atrophicans inversa
   JEB progressiva
   JEB with pyloric atresia ($\alpha_6\beta_4$ integrin)
   Generalized atrophic benign EB (GABEB) (BP Ag II)
   Cicatricial JEB

Dermolytic or dystrophic (*sublamina densa*) (collagen VII)
   Dominant forms
   Dystrophic EB, hyperplastic variant (Cockayne-Touraine)
      Dystrophic EB, albopapuloid variant (Pasini)
      Bart's syndrome (congenital localized skin defects)
      Transient bullous dermolysis of the newborn
      Acrokeratotic poikiloderma (Weary-Kindler)

Recessive forms
　Generalized (gravis or mitis)
　Localized
　Inverse

Odom RB, James WD, Berger TG. Andrews' Diseases of the Skin, 9th ed. Philadelphia: W.B. Saunders Co. 2000: p. 693.

Structure and Function of the Skin

Plasma membrane   BP-Ag 1 (BP230)
                       BP-Ag 2 (BP180; type XVII collagen)
                       Transmembrane (NC16A domain)
                       Plectin
                       $\alpha_6\beta_4$ integrin (TM protein of HD),
                       $\alpha_3\beta_1$
Anchoring filaments Laminin V/VI

Lamina lucida   Laminin I
                       Laminin V (kalinin, epiligrin, nicein)

Lamina densa   Collagen V   Heparin sulfate
                       Entactin/nidogen   Laminin 6 and 10

Sublamina densa   Anchoring fibrils
                       Collagen VII
                       Linkin, Tenascin

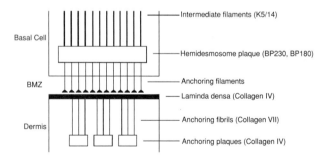

AJCC Melanoma TNM Classification

T classification	Thickness (mm)	Ulceration
Tx	1° tumor cannot be assessed	
T0	No evidence of 1° tumor	
TIS	Carcinoma in situ	
T 1	≤1.0	a: no ulceration; level II/III
		b: ulceration or level IV/V
T 2	1.01–2.0	a: no ulceration
		b: ulceration
T 3	2.01–4.0	a: no ulceration
		b: with ulceration
T 4	>4.0	a: no ulceration
		b: with ulceration

N classification	Metastatic nodes	Nodal metastatic mass
Nx	Regional nodes cannot be assessed	
N0	No regional lymphadenopathy	
N2L	Satellite or in-transit metastasis without nodal metastases	
N 1	1 node	a: micrometastasis[1]
		b: macrometastasis[2]
N 2	2–3 nodes or intralymphatic regional mets without nodal mets	a: micrometastasis[1]
		b: macrometastasis[2]
		c: satellite/in transit without nodal

N classification	Metastatic nodes	Nodal metastatic mass
N 3	≥4 metastatic nodes or matted nodes, or in transit met(s)/satellites with metastatic node(s)	

M classification	Metastases (site)
Mx	Distant metastasis cannot be assessed
M0	No distant metastasis
M1a	Distal skin, subcutaneous/distant nodes
M1b	Lung
M1c	All other visceral + normal LDH
	Any distant metastases + ↑ LDH

[1] Micrometastases diagnosed after sentinel or elective lymphadenectomy
[2] Macrometastases defined as clinically detectable nodal metastases confirmed by therapeutic lymphadenectomy or when nodal metastasis exhibits gross extracapsular extension.

Used with permission (Balch CM et al. Final version of the American Joint Committee on Cancer Staging System for cutaneous melanoma. *J Clin Oncol* 2001;19: pp. 3635–3648.)

AJCC Staging for Cutaneous Melanoma

	Clinical staging			Pathologic staging		
	T	N	M	T	N	M
0	Tis	N0	M0	Tis	N0	M0
IA	T1a	N0	M0	T1a	N0	M0
IB	T1b	N0	M0	T1b	N0	M0
	T2a	N0	M0	T2a	N0	M0
IIA	T2b	N0	M0	T2b	N0	M0
	T3a	N0	M0	T3a	N0	M0
IIB	T3b	N0	M0	T3b	N0	M0
	T4a	N0	M0	T4a	N0	M0
IIC	T4b	N0	M0	T4b	N0	M0
III	Any T	N1	M0			
		N2				
		N3				
IIIA	T1–4a	N1a	M0	T1–4a	N1a	M0
	T1–4a	N2	M0	T1–4a	N2a	M0
IIIB	T1–4b			T1–4b	N1a	M0
				T1–4b	N2a	M0
				T1–4a	N1b	M0
				T1–4a	N2b	M0
				T1–4a/b	N2c	M0
IIIC				T1–4b	N1b	M0
				T1–4b	N2b	M0
				Any T	N3	M0
IV	Any T	Any N	Any M1	Any T	Any N	Any M1

Used with permission (Balch CM et al. Final version of the American Joint Committee on Cancer Staging System for cutaneous melanoma. *J Clin Oncol* 2001;19: pp. 3635–3648.)

Treatment and Survival of Malignant Melanoma

Guidelines for surgical management[1]

Thickness (mm)	Margins (cm)
In situ	0.5
≤1	1
1–2	1–2
2–4	2
4	2–3

5 year survival rates of pathologically staged patients

	Ta: nonulcerated (%)	*Tb: ulcerated (%)*
IA	95	
IB	89	91
IIA	79	77
IIB	67	63
IIC		45
IIIA	67	
IIIB	54	52
IIIC	28	24

[1] Treatment with Mohs micrographic surgery is also a therapeutic option. Zitelli JA, Brown CD, Hanusa BH. Surgical margins for excision of primary cutaneous melanoma. *J Am Acad Dermatol* 1997; 37: 422–429.

Balch CM, Buzaid A, Atkins MB et al. Final version of AJCC Staging System for Cutaneous Melanoma. *J Clin Oncol* 2001; 19: 3635–3648.

Clark and Breslow Staging of Melanoma

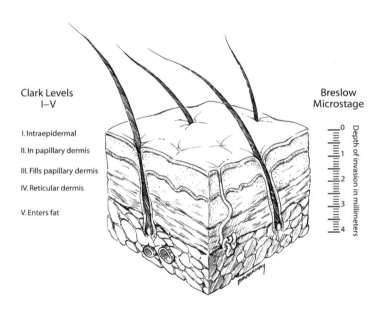

Clark Levels
I–V

I. Intraepidermal

II. In papillary dermis

III. Fills papillary dermis

IV. Reticular dermis

V. Enters fat

Breslow
Microstage

Depth of invasion in millimeters

0
1
2
3
4

AJCC Staging for Basal Cell Carcinoma and Cutaneous Squamous Cell Carcinoma

T classification

TX   Primary tumor cannot be assessed

T0   No evidence of primary tumor

Tis Carcinoma in situ

T1   Tumor ≤ 2 cm

T2   Tumor >2 cm but <5 cm

T3   Tumor >5 cm

T4   Invades deep extradermal structures

*with multiple simultaneous tumors, the tumor with highest T category is classified and number of separate tumors is indicated in parentheses.

N classification

NX   Regional lymph nodes cannot be assessed

N0   No regional lymph node metastasis

N1   Regional lymph node metastasis

M classification

MX   Distant metastasis cannot be assessed

M0   No distant metastasis

M1   Distant mestastasis

Staging

Stage 0   Tis, N0, M0

Stage I   T1, N0, M0

Stage II   T2, N0, M0

               T3, N0, M0

Stage III T4, N0, M0

               Any T, N1, M0

Stage IV   Any T, any N, M1

Histologic Grading of Cutaneous Squamous Cell Carcinoma

Broder's grade	Differentiation	Microscopic appearance
I	Well differentiated	>75% mature keratinocytes
II	Moderately well differentiated	50–75% mature keratinocytes
III	Poorly differentiated	25–50% mature keratinocytes
IV	Anaplastic/ Pleomorphic	<25% mature keratinocytes

Lohmann CM, Solomon AR. Clinicopathologic variants of cutaneous squamous cell carcinoma. *Adv Anatom Pathol* 2001; 8: 27–36.

CTCL (TNMB) Classification and Staging

T0   Nondiagnostic

T1   Limited patch/plaque (<10% total skin surface)

T2   Generalized patch/plaque ($\geq$10% total skin surface)

T3   Tumors ($\geq$1 cutaneous tumor)

T4   Erythroderma ($\pm$ patches, plaques, tumors)

N0   Lymph nodes clinically uninvolved

N1   Lymph nodes enlarged; no histologic involvement

N2   Lymph nodes clinically uninvolved; histologic involvement

N3   Lymph nodes enlarged; histologic involvement

M0   No visceral involvement

M1   Visceral involvement (confirmed with pathology)

B0   No circulating atypical/Sézary cells (<5% of lymphocytes) (<1000 Sézary cells [CD4+ CD7−]/ml)

B1   Circulating atypical/Sézary cells ($\geq$5% of lymphocytes) ($\geq$1000 Sézary cells [CD4+ CD7−]/ml)

Stage	T	N	M
IA	1	0	0
IB	2	0	0
IIA	1–2	1	0
IIB	3	0–1	0
IIIA	4	0	0
IIIB	4	1	0
IVA	1–4	2–3	0
IVB	1–4	0–3	1

Note: Due to automated blood counts, most often see Sezary cell count from peripheral blood flow cytometry reports.

Fung MA et al. Practical evaluation and management of cutaneous lymphoma. *J Am Acad Dermatol* 2002; 46: 325.

Toxic Epidermal Necrolysis (TEN) Protocol

A   Admit to ICU

D   Diagnosis: Toxic Epidermal Necrolysis (TEN)

C   Condition

V   Vitals

A   Activity: bed rest

A   Allergies

N   Nursing

     air/fluid bed; pulmonary toilet

     leave unbroken blisters intact; gentle debridement
       of raw skin

     biologic dressings over denuded skin; cover with gauze
       daily recording of % skin detached, % involved

D   Diet: consult nutrition; NG tube or TPN if cannot
     tolerate NG

I   IVF: IV at site of intact epidermis (cc/hr adj. by UO and
     RFTs)

S   Specific medications

    IVIG (0.75–1 mg/kg/d × 3–5 days (tot. 4 g/kg); monitor
    IgA level

     erythromycin opthalmic ointment q2 hr

     anticoagulants (heparin, lovenox)

     antibiotics as indicated ($\uparrow$ culture titers, $\downarrow$ temp or WBC)

S   Symptomatic medications

     MSO_4 iv/po; midazolam prn and for dressing changes

     prophylactic antacid

E   Extra studies and consults

     Consult critical care and ophthalmology

     CXR: baseline photographs

L   Labs: CBC, CMP, CPK, PT/PTT, amylase, lipase
        stat IgA level (follow WBC and BUN qd)
        wound swab cultures q2 days
        blood cultures prior to starting antibiotics (over intact
            skin)
        stat skin biopsy

Therapeutics

Intravenous Immunoglobulin (IVIG)

Mechanism: blockade of reticuloendothelial fragment crystallizable (Fc) receptors, impedance of complement-mediated damage, alteration of cytokine/cytokine antagonist levels, ↓ circulating Ab, elimination of pathogens

Metabolism:

Excretion:

Dosing: 0.5–1 g/kg/day × 1–3 days (variable)

Pregnancy cat.: Not listed

Side effects: injection reaction (≤1 hr); headache, flushing, chills, myalgia, wheezing, back pain, nausea, hypotension, anaphylaxis with IgA deficiency, thrombosis

Monitoring: IgA level (70–400 mg/dL for adults)

Notes: produced by mature plasma cells

composed predominantly of IgG

caution with IgA deficiency

SCORTEN classification (see next page)

Trent JT et al. Analysis of intravenous immmunoglobulin for the treatment of toxic epidermal necrolysis using SCORTEN. *Arch Dermatol* 2003; 139: 39–43.

Bystryn JC et al. Treatment of pemphigus vulgaris with intravenous immunoglobulin. *J Am Acad Dermatol* 2002; 47: 358–362.

Sheehan DJ, Lesher JL. Deep venous thrombosis after high-dose intravenous immunoglobulin in the treatment of pemphigus vulgaris. *Cutis* 2004; 73: 403–406.

SCORTEN

SCORTEN risk factors (presence of each counts as 1):
- Age >40 yrs
- Malignancy
- BSA involved >10%
- HR >120 bpm
- $HCO3^-$ <20 mEq/L
- Glu >252 mg/dl
- BUN >28 mg/dl

SCORTEN	Mortality rate (%)
0–1	3.2
2	12.1
3	35.3
4	58.3
≥5	90

Bastuji-Garin, Fouchard N, Mertocchi M, Roujeau JC, Revuz J, Wolkenstein P. SCORTEN: A severity-of-illness score for toxic epidermal necrolysis. *J Invest Dermatol* 2000; 115: 149–153.

Systemic Retinoids

Isotretinoin (Accutane)

Mechanism: activate nuclear receptors; regulates transcription

Metabolism: hepatic (oxidation and chain shortening)

Excretion: bile and urine

Dosing: 0.5–1 mg/kg/day × 16–20 weeks

Pregnancy cat.: X

Side effects: multiple (teratogenic)

potential risk of depression

(controversial) mucocutaneous dryness/side effects musculoskeletal aches; alopecia

Monitoring: β-HCG, lipid profile, LFT, RFT, CBC

Notes: recommend ≥120 mg/kg over 5-month period

calculation: weight (kg) × 3 = total # of 40 mg caps

avoid elective surgery

Acitretin (Soriatane)

Mechanism: multiple (alteration of sebaceous glands)

Metabolism: hepatic (isomerization and chain shortening)

Excretion: bile and urine

Dosing: 25–50 mg po qd

Pregnancy cat.: X

Side effects: multiple (teratogenic); mucocutaneous reaction, musculoskeletal, telogen effluvium

Monitoring: β-HCG, lipid profile, LFT, RFT, CBC

Notes   Pt should not become pregnant, drink
                          ethanol or have cosmetic surgery (risk of
                          hypertrophic scarring) for ≥ 2 years

Nguyen EQH, Wolverton SE. ed. In: Wolverton SE, ed. Comprehensive Dermatologic Drug Therapy. Philadelphia: W. B. Saunders Co. 2001: p. 269.

Systemic Antibacterials

Doxycycline (tetracycline)

Mechanism:	inhibits bacterial protein synthesis (binds 30S)
Metabolism:	hepatic (minimal)
Excretion:	GI tract
Dosing:	100 mg po qd to bid
Pregnancy cat.:	**D**
Side effects:	photosensitivity
Monitoring:	none
Notes:	only tetracycline acceptable for use in renal failure
	well absorbed with food intake
	not recommended <9 years of age (stains teeth)

Minocycline (tetracycline)

Mechanism:	inhibits bacterial protein synthesis (binds 30S)
Metabolism:	hepatic (partially)
Excretion:	urine
Dosing:	50–100 mg po qd to bid
Pregnancy cat.:	**D**
Side effects:	hypersensitivity reactions
	drug-induced lupus erythematosus dizziness
Monitoring:	none
Notes:	well absorbed with food intake

Tetracycline (tetracycline)

Mechanism:	inhibits bacterial protein synthesis (binds 30S)

Metabolism:	hepatic (partially)
Excretion:	urine
Dosing:	250–500 mg po bid
Pregnancy cat.:	**D**
Side effects:	hypersensitivity reactions
Monitoring:	none
Notes:	not well absorbed with food intake
	do not administer to children ≤8 years of age (stains teeth)
	take 1 hour before or 2 hours after meals
	tetracycline may have some MMP inhibitor effect (hence use in BP)

Erythromycin (macrolide)

Mechanism:	bind 50S: inhibits RNA-dependent protein synthesis
Metabolism:	hepatic
Excretion:	feces and urine
Dosing:	250–500 mg po qid (bid for acne)
Pregnancy cat.:	**B**
Side effects:	hypersensitivity reactions; nausea; diarrhea
Monitoring:	none
Notes:	inhibits cytochrome P-450 (drug interactions)
	avoid erythromycin estolate in pregnancy (hepatitis)
	avoid with cytochrome P-450 3A inhibitors – combination can lead to increased erythromycin and sudden cardiac death

Azithromycin (macrolide [azalide])

Mechanism:	bind 50S: inhibits RNA-dependent protein synthesis
Metabolism:	hepatic (unlike clarithromycin)
Excretion:	feces and urine
Dosing:	250 mg 2–3×/week (acne) or 5 day dose-pack
Pregnancy cat.:	**B**
Side effects:	hypersensitivity reactions
Monitoring:	none
Notes:	does not affect cytochrome P-450 system

Dicloxacillin (β-lactamase resistant penicillin)

Mechanism:	inhibit bacterial cell wall synthesis
Metabolism:	hepatic (partially)
Excretion:	urine
Dosing:	250–500 mg po qid
Pregnancy cat.:	**B**
Side effects:	hypersensitivity reactions; GI effects
Monitoring:	none
Notes:	best taken on an empty stomach

Cephalexin (cephalosporin)

Mechanism:	inhibit penicillin-binding proteins
Metabolism:	other
Excretion:	urine
Dosing:	250 mg po qid
Pregnancy cat.:	**B**
Side effects:	GI toxicity; hypersensitivity reactions
Monitoring:	none

Notes: ~5% penicillin allergy cross-reactivity

absorbed in upper intestine

serum half life 1–2 hours (hence qid dosing)

Ciprofloxacin (quinolone)

Mechanism: inhibits DNA gyrase (bacterial

topoisomerase II)

Metabolism: hepatic

Excretion: renal (feces and urine)

Dosing: 500–750 mg po bid

Pregnancy cat.:   **C**

Side effects: hypersensitivity reactions; nausea; diarrhea;

vomiting; headache; dizziness; sleep

disturbances

Monitoring: none

Notes: most effective against gram (−) organisms

active against *Pseudomonas aeruginosa*

associated with decreased seizure

threshold evening dosing has decreased

phototoxic potential

decreased bioavailability with Al,

Mg, Fe, Zn

excellent for multiresistant gram (−)

organisms

risk of tendon rupture (especially children)

Levofloxacin (quinolone)

Mechanism: inhibits DNA gyrase (bacterial

topoisomerase II)

Metabolism: hepatic

Excretion: urine

Dosing: 500–750 mg po qd

Pregnancy cat.:	**C**
Side effects:	hypersensitivity reactions; nausea; diarrhea; vomiting; headache; dizziness; sleep disturbances; arthropathy
Monitoring:	none
Notes:	most effective against gram (−) organisms active against *Pseudomonas aeruginosa* associated with decreased seizure threshold decreased bioavailability with Al, Mg, Fe, Zn excellent for multiresistant gram (−) organisms risk of tendon rupture (especially children)

Trimethoprim-Sulfamethoxazole (TMP:SMX = 1:5)

Mechanism:	inhibits 2-step conversion of folate to tetrahydrofolate in bacteria; disrupts nucleic acid synthesis
Metabolism:	hepatic
Excretion:	urine
Dosing:	1 tab po bid (DS: 160 mg TMP/800 mg SMX)
Pregnancy cat.:	**C**
Side effects:	hypersensitivity reactions; infrequent risk of Stevens–Johnson syndrome; GI toxicity; increased risk of maculopapular eruptions in HIV patients
Monitoring:	none
Notes:	avoid in patients taking methotrexate caution in patients taking coumadin increased risk of drug reaction with family history

Rifampin

Mechanism:	inhibits DNA-dependent RNA polymerase
Metabolism:	hepatic
Excretion:	feces
Dosing:	10–20 mg/kg po qd (max 600 mg/day)
Pregnancy cat.:	**C**
Side effects:	reddish-orange body fluids; hypersensitivity
Monitoring:	monitor transaminase levels for use >7–10 days
Notes:	take on empty stomach 1 hr before/2 hr after meal
	potential induction of hepatic microsomal enzymes
	should only be used in conjunction with another gram (+) agent (NEVER use alone)
	poor gram (−) coverage
	decreases efficacy of oral contraceptives (strong CYP3A4 inducer)
	usually used by Infectious Disease specialists
	part of ROM (rifampin, ofloxacin, minocycline) therapy for leprosy

Clindamycin

Mechanism:	binds 50S → inhibits protein synthesis via blocking transpeptidation
Metabolism:	hepatic
Excretion:	other
Dosing:	150–300 mg po bid to tid

Pregnancy cat.:	**B**
Side effects:	antibiotic-associated colitis (rarely)
Monitoring:	none
Notes:	poor gram $(-)$ activity
	neuromuscular blocking properties may
	enhance other neuromuscular agents
	good anaerobic coverage

Sadick NS. Systemic Antibacterial Agents. In: Wolverton SE. ed., ed. Comprehensive Dermatologic Drug Therapy. Philadelphia: W. B. Saunders Co. 2001: p. 28.

Ray WA, Murray KT, Meredith S et al. Oral erythromycin and the risk of sudden death from cardiac causes. *N Engl J Med* 2004; 351: 1089–1096.

Yee CL, Duffy C, Gerbino PG et al. Tendon or joint disorders in children after treatment with fluoroquinolones or azithromycin. *Pediatr Infect Dis J* 2002; 21: 525–529.

Topical Antimicrobials

Bacitracin

- inhibits bacterial cell wall synthesis – inhibits peptidoglycan synthesis
- gram (+): *S. aureus, S. pneumoniae, Neisseria, H. influenzae, T. pallidum*
- gram (−): minimal coverage
- SE: contact sensitization, rare anaphylaxis

Mupirocin (Bactroban)

- inhibits bacterial RNA and protein synthesis (isoleucyl tDNA synthetase)
- gram (+):   Staphylococci (MRSA), Streptococci
- gram (−):   some gram (−) cocci
- SE: local irritant
- does not cross-react with other topical antimicrobials
- renal toxicity when used on large denuded areas
- uncommon contact sensitization

Neomycin

- inhibits protein synthesis (binds 30S subunit)
- gram (+): good coverage vs. *S. aureus* (weak for *Strep*)
- gram (−): yes
- SE: ototoxic and nephrotoxic; contact sensitization; virtually always used in combination

Polymyxin B

- antibacterial via surface detergent-like mechanisms
- gram (+): no activity
- gram (−): *Proteus, Pseudomonas, Serratia*
- SE: rare contact sensitization

Spann CT et al. Topical antibacterial agents for wound care: A primer. *Dermatol Surg* 2003; 29: 620–626.

Systemic Antifungals

Terbinafine (allylamine)

Mechanism:	inhibits squalene epoxidase (↑squalene and impairs ergosterol synthesis)
Metabolism:	hepatic (80%); fecal (20%) −15 metabolites
Excretion:	renal
Dosing:	250 mg po qd (12 wks – toenails; 6 wks – fingernails)
	125 mg po qd (20–40 kg)
	62.5 mg po qd (<20 kg)
Pregnancy cat.:	**B** (excreted in breast milk; not rec. in pregnancy)
Side effects:	headache, GI symptoms, morbilliform rash, dysguesia
Monitoring:	LFTs (transaminases) and CBC after 6 wks
Notes:	less effective for *Candida* than azole antifungals
	caution with concomitant doxepin due to terbinafine CYP 2D6 interaction
	caution with renal insufficiency/hepatic dysfunction
	safe and effective in children for same duration
	use $\frac{1}{2}$ dose with elevated creatine

Itraconazole (triazole)

Mechanism:	inhibits lanosterol 14-a demethylase (inhibits lanosterol → ergosterol)
Metabolism:	hepatic (side-chain hydroxylation to hydroxyitraconazole)
Excretion:	renal (urine 35%; feces 54%)

Dosing: 200 mg po bid × 1 week/month (pulse regimen)

(2 pulses for fingernails; 3–4 pulses for toenails)

Pregnancy cat.: **C** (excreted in breast milk)

Side effects: headache, GI symptoms, morbilliform rash

Monitoring: LFTs after 4 wks (some do not check)

Notes: highest po bioavailability with full meal/carbonated

safe and effective in children

CYP 3A4 inhibitor (less than terbinafine)

Ketoconazole

Mechanism: inhibits lanosterol 14-a demethylase

Metabolism: hepatic (side-chain hydroxylation)

Excretion: renal

Dosing: 200–400 mg po qd

Pregnancy cat.: **C** (excreted in breast milk)

Side effects: headache, GI symptoms, morbilliform rash

Monitoring: LFT after 2 weeks

Notes: highest po bioavailability with full meal

caution with hepatic dysfunction

T. versicolor dosing: 400 mg/day qweek × 2 weeks

Fluconazole

Mechanism: inhibits fungal lanosterol 14-a demethylase

Metabolism: hepatic (no significant 1st-pass hepatic metabolism)

Excretion: renal

Dosing:	150 mg po qweek (vulvovaginal candidiasis)
	300–450 mg po qweek (off-label, onychomycosis)
Pregnancy cat.:	**C**
Side effects:	few adverse effects
Monitoring:	usually not needed
Notes:	penetrates into CSF well
	excellent po bioavailability (>90%)
	no need to renal dose for single
	dose multiple drug interactions (cytochrome P-450)
	minimal CYP 3A4 inhibition at doses <300 mg qd
	CYP 2C9 inhibition (extreme caution with warfarin)

Griseofulvin

Mechanism:	inhibits microtubule formation
Metabolism:	hepatic
Excretion:	renal
Dosing:	
Adult:	250 mg po bid
Pediatric:	20 mg/kg po qd (microsize and ultramicrosize)
Pregnancy cat.:	**C**
Side effects:	granulocytopenia, hepatotoxicity, urticaria
Monitoring:	none

Notes: absorption improved with fatty meal
                   shake liquid before dispersing
                   decreases efficacy of oral contraceptives
                   possible cross-reactivity in penicillin
                   allergic patient

lb	kg	ml (125/5)	tspn
20	9.1	7.3	1.5
25	11.4	9.1	1.8
30	13.6	10.9	2.2
35	15.9	12.7	2.5
40	18.2	14.5	2.9
45	20.5	16.4	3.3
50	22.7	18.2	3.6
55	25.0	20.0	4.0
60	27.3	21.8	4.4
65	29.5	23.6	4.7
70	31.8	25.5	5.1
75	34.1	27.3	5.5
80	36.4	29.1	5.8
85	38.6	30.9	6.2
90	40.9	32.7	6.5
95	43.2	34.5	6.9
100	45.5	36.4	7.3

Phillips RM and Rosen T. Topical antifungal agents. In: Wolverton SE. ed. Comprehensive Dermatologic Drug Therapy. Philadelphia: W. B. Saunders Co. 2001: p. 55.

Systemic Antivirals

Acyclovir

Mechanism: inhibits viral DNA polymerase (requires thymidine kinase)

Metabolism: (no hepatic microsomal metabolism)

Excretion: renal

Dosing: *genital herpes (1st)*: 200 mg po 5×/day × 10 days

genital herpes (rec): 200 mg po 5×/day × 5 days

genital herpes (suppressive): 400 mg po bid

herpes zoster: 800 mg po 5×/day × 7–10 days

HSV infection: 5 mg/kg iv q8° × 7 days

HSV encephalitis: 10 mg/kg iv q8° × 10 days

acute varicella: 800 mg po qid × 5 days

disseminated HSV: 10 mg/kg iv q8° × 7 days

HSV keratitis: 400 mg po 5×/day

herpes zoster ophthalmicus: 800 mg po 5×/day

Pregnancy cat.: B

Side effects: leukopenia, thrombocytopenia (rare with po), renal (occurs with rapid iv infusion)

Monitoring: none

Notes: generally well-tolerated

Valacyclovir

Mechanism: inhibits viral DNA polymerase (requires thymidine kinase)

Metabolism:	no hepatic microsomal metabolism
Excretion:	feces and urine
Dosing:	genital herpes (1st): 1000 mg po bid × 10 days
	genital herpes (rec): 500 mg po bid × 3 days
	genital herpes (prophylaxis): 500–1000 mg po qd
	herpes zoster: 1000 mg po tid × 7 days
	oral herpes: 2 g po bid × 1 day
Pregnancy cat.:	**B**
Side effects:	nausea, headaches
Notes:	po bioavailability 3–5 × that of acyclovir
	prodrug of acyclovir

Famciclovir

Mechanism:	inhibits viral DNA polymerase (requires thymidine kinase)
Metabolism:	no hepatic microsomal metabolism
Excretion:	urine
Dosing:	genital herpes (1st): 250 mg po tid × 7 days
	genital herpes (rec): 125 mg po bid × 5 days
	genital herpes (prophylaxis): 250 mg po bid
	herpes zoster: 500 mg po q8° × 7 days
Pregnancy cat.:	**B**
Side effects:	nausea, headaches
Notes:	prodrug of penciclovir

Evans TY, Straten MRV, Carrasco DA, Carlton S, Tyring SK. Systemic Antiviral Agents. In: Wolverton SE. ed. Comprehensive Dermatologic Drug Therapy. Philadelphia: W. B. Saunders Co. 2001: p. 85.

Methotrexate

Mechanism:	inhibits dihydrofolate reductase (S phase specific)
Metabolism:	hepatic (triphasic reduction)
Excretion:	renal
Dosing:	2.5–20 mg po qweek (can also dose iv or im)
Pregnancy cat.:	X
Side effects:	hepatotoxicity, pulmonary toxicity, GI, pancytopenia, teratogenic, tibial osteopathy
Monitoring:	CBC, LFT, RFT, hepatitis profile (baseline) liver biopsy > 2 g without liver disease/ethanol use and then repeat at intervals
Notes:	test dose of 5–10 mg qd (CBC, LFTs 1 week later)
	may divide dose q12 hr × 3 doses for nausea
	may supplement folate 1 mg po qD for nausea
	antidote for overdose: folinic acid
	unaffected by food intake in adults
	interacts with weak acids (probenecid, salicylate, sulfonamide)
	↓ renal function increases risk of hepatic and hematologic toxicity

Roenigk Classification of Liver Biopsies

Grade	Histology	Action
I	Normal; mild fatty infiltration	May continue
II	Fatty infiltration (mod to severe)	May continue
IIIA	Fibrosis (mild)	May continue but need liver biopsy after 6 mo
IIIB	Fibrosis (moderate to severe)	Discontinue
IV	Cirrhosis	Discontinue

Callen JP, Kulp-Shorten CL, Wolverton SE. Methotrexate. In: Wolverton SE. ed. Comprehensive Dermatologic Drug Therapy. Philadelphia: W. B. Saunders Co. 2001: p. 147.

Zachariae H. Liver biopsies and methotrexate: A time for reconsideration? *J Amer Acad Dermatol* 2000; 42: 531–534.

Dapsone

Mechanism:	inhibits myeloperoxidase; affects neutrophil chemotaxis; inhibits folic acid pathway
Metabolism:	hepatic (N-acetylation and N-hydroxylation)
Excretion:	hepatic and renal
Dosing:	begin 25–50 mg po qd; increase to 100–200 mg
Pregnancy cat.:	C
Side effects:	hemolysis, methemoglobinemia, leukopenia, agranulocytosis, distal motor neuropathy
Monitoring:	Baseline: G6PD, UA, RFT
	Routine: CBC, reticulocyte count
Notes:	crosses placenta and excreted in breast milk
	hemolysis can occur in nursing infants
	metabolism inhibited by cimetidine
	well absorbed from gut
	drug of choice for dermatitis herpetiformis
	sulfapyradine may be alternate
	can reduce dapsone-induced methemoglobinemia by co-administration of cimetidine

Hall RP. Dapsone. In: Wolverton SE, ed. Comprehensive Dermatologic Drug Therapy. Philadelphia: W. B. Saunders Co. 2001: p. 230.

Systemic Immunomodulators

Azathioprine (Imuran)

Mechanism:	inhibits DNA/RNA synthesis/repair
	alters T and B-cell function,
	decreases number of Langerhans cells/APCs
Metabolism:	i. anabolized by HGPRT $\to$ active 6-thioguanine
	ii. catabolized by thiopurine methyltransferase
	iii. catabolized by xanthine oxidase (XO)
Excretion:	Negligible (virtually completely metabolized)
Dosing (TPMT):	High (>19 U) $\to$ $\leq$2.5 mg/kg/day
	Medium (13.7–19 U) $\to$ $\leq$1.5 mg/kg/day
	Low (5–13.7 U) $\to$ $\leq$0.5 mg/kg/day
	<5.0 U $\to$ no treatment
Pregnancy cat.:	**D**
Side effects:	pancytopenia (increased risk with $\downarrow$ TPMT), immunosuppression carcinogenesis (non-Hodgkin's, squamous cell carcinoma)
	opportunistic infections
	GI side effects
	hypersensitivity syndrome
Monitoring:	Baseline: CBC, LFT, RFT, β-HCG (CBC, AST, ALT q1 mo $\times$ 3 then q 2 mo)
Notes:	XO pathway can be inhibited by allopurinol
	Lower azathioprine dose by 75% with allopurinol

TMPT gene (6p22.3) – autosomal codominant

Interactions: allopurinol, captopril, warfarin, pancuronium

Cyclosporine (Neoral)

Mechanism: inhibits calcineurin with resultant $\downarrow$NFAT-1 and IL-2

Metabolism: hepatic (CYP 3A4)

Excretion: hepatobiliary (neither dialysis nor renal failure significantly alters drug clearance)

Dosing: 3–5 mg/kg/day

Pregnancy cat.: **C**

Side effects: nephrotoxicity, hypertension, neurotoxicity, tremors, hypertrichosis; hyperlipidemia

Monitoring: LFT, RFT, CBC, lipid profile, K^+, Mg^{++} blood pressure

Notes: avoid concomitant use of grapefruit juice (apple or orange juice acceptable to use)

avoid concomitant use of erythromycin, ketoconazole or other CYP 3A4 inhibitors

decrease dose (0.5–1 mg/kg/day) if creatinine $\uparrow$ by 30% from baseline (recheck in 2 weeks)

sequential psoriasis therapy – use for 3–4 months

consider sequential use with acitretin

multiple drug interactions (always check potential interactions prior to use)

cannot use with aminophylline

$$Creatinine(clearance) = \frac{(140 - age) \times (wt(kg))}{Cr(mg/100ml) \times 72} \times 0.85(woman)$$

Koo JYM, Lee CS, Maloney JE. Cyclosporine and related drugs. In: Wolverton SE. ed. Comprehensive Dermatologic Drug Therapy. Philadelphia: W. B. Saunders Co. 2001: p. 205.

Cytotoxic Agents

Cyclophosphamide (Cytoxan)

Mechanism:	alkylating agent (cell cycle non-specific)
	depresses B-cell function > T-cell function
Metabolism:	hepatic
Excretion:	hepatic; renal (10–20%)
Dosing:	1–3 mg/kg/day (50–200 mg/day) (single am
	dose)
Pregnancy cat.:	C
Side effects:	carcinogenic (including bladder carcinoma)
	hemorrhagic cystitis
Monitoring:	WBC (caution if <4000/mm^3)
	Granulocyte count (caution <2000/mm^3)
	leukocyte nadir occurs at 8–12 days
	urinalysis
Notes:	converted to acrolein (active metabolite)
	acrolein is source of bladder toxicity
	↑ po fluid intake to avoid hemorrhagic cystitis
	D/C with hematuria

Mycophenolate mofetil (Cellcept)

Mechanism:	inhibits inosine monophosphate dehydrogenase
	inhibits de novo purine synthesis
Metabolism:	hepatic (hydrolyzed to active mycophenolate acid)
Excretion:	renal (93% urine; 6% feces; skin minimal)
Dosing:	1–2 g/day (may use up to 3 g/day in autoimmune skin diseases)
Pregnancy cat.:	C
Side effects:	GI toxicity (dose-dependent); ↑herpes zoster
Monitoring:	CBC with diff.; (caution if WBC <4000–4500/mm^3) LFTs
Notes:	well-tolerated
	T and B cells cannot use alternate salvage guanosine synthesis pathway → depend critically on de novo synthesis of purines
	competes with salicylate and furosemide and albumin no nephrotoxicity (hepatotoxicity only rarely)

Pan TD, McDonald CJ. Cytotoxic agents. In: Wolverton SE, ed. Comprehensive Dermatologic Drug Therapy. Philadelphia: W. B. Saunders Co. 2001: p. 180.

Menon K and Shipack J. Mycophenolate mofetil for dermatology. *Contemp Dermatol* 2003; 1: 1–8.

Antimalarial Agents

Hydroxychloroquine (Plaquenil)

Mechanism:	unknown
Metabolism:	unknown
Excretion:	urine and/or biliary
Dosing:	200–400 mg po qd; max chronic dose 6.5 mg/kg/d
Pregnancy cat.:	C
Side effects:	ocular toxicity, hematologic, GI, neuromusc, skin
Monitoring:	G6PD (baseline), CBC, chemistry profile; LFTs, eye exam yearly
Notes:	tendency to worsen psoriasis

Chloroquine (Aralen)

Mechanism:	unknown
Metabolism:	unknown
Dosing:	250–500 mg po qd; max chronic dose 4 mg/kg/d
Pregnancy cat.:	C
Side effects:	ocular toxicity, hematologic, GI, neuromusc, skin
Monitoring:	G6PD (baseline), CBC, chemistry profile; LFTs, eye exam yearly
Notes:	may induce pruritus

Quinacrine (Atabrine)

Mechanism:	unknown
Metabolism:	unknown

Dosing: 100–200 mg po qd; max chronic dose
                       6.5 mg/kg/d

Pregnancy cat.:   **C**

Side effects: hematologic, GI, neuromusc, skin yellowing

Monitoring: G6PD (baseline), CBC, chemistry profile;
                       LFTs

Notes: no significant potential for retinopathy
                       may add to either of above 2 at
                       100 mg/day *without* ↑ risk of
                       retinotoxicity

Callen JP, Camisa C. Antimalarial agents. In: Wolverton SE, ed. Comprehensive Dermatologic Drug Therapy. Philadelphia: W. B. Saunders Co. 2001: p. 147.

Biologics

Terminology:
- ximab
- zimab
- umab

- chimeric molecule
- humanized molecule
- human sequence generated via monoclonal Ab

- cept
- receptor fusion protein fused to segment of Ab

Adalimumab (Humira®)

Mechanism:	inhibits β receptor (TNF-α)
Excretion:	urine
Dosing:	40 mg SC q other week
Pregnancy cat.:	**B**
Side effects:	rare demyelinating disorders
	opportunistic infections
	malignancy
Monitoring:	baseline PPD
Notes:	indicated for rheumatoid arthritis
	recombinant human IgG1 monoclonal antibody against TNF-α
	can use with methotrexate
	no pediatric studies at this time
	800–4HUMIRA

Alefacept (Amevive®)

Mechanism:	blocks LFA-3 and inhibits CD45RO+ (memory)T-cells

Excretion:	
Dosing:	15 mg IM q week × 12 weeks
Pregnancy cat.:	**B**
Side effects:	injection site reactions; T-cell depletion; infection; malignancy; lymphopenia; serious infections
Monitoring:	CD 4 at baseline and q week (D/C if <250)
Notes:	FDA approval for psoriasis
	not approved for pediatric use
	repeat cycle may be given 12 weeks after first
	866-AMEVIVE

Efaluzimab (Raptiva®)

Mechanism:	inhibits CD11a
Excretion:	degraded
Dosing:	0.7 mg/kg test dose (1 week washout)
	1 mg/kg SC q week (max 200 mg)
Pregnancy cat.:	**C**
Side effects:	HA, chills, nausea, fever, myalgia, rebound
Monitoring:	Recommend PLT count baseline, 1st 3 months, then quarterly
Notes:	potential for rebound upon discontinuation
	recombinant humanized IgG1 kappa monoclonal antibody against CD11a
	may cause transient lymphocytosis
	FDA approved for psoriasis
	not approved for pediatric use
	rapid onset of action (2–4 weeks)
	877-RAPTIVA

Etanercept (Enbrel®)

Mechanism:	inhibits TNF-$\alpha\beta$ (transmembrane)
Excretion:	urine
Dosing:	50 mg SC q week
Pregnancy cat.:	**B**
Side effects:	injection site reactions; CNS disorders; hematologic abn
Monitoring:	baseline PPD
Notes:	approved for pediatric use
	FDA approval for psoriasis, psoriatic arthritis, rheumatoid arthritis, ankylosing spondylitis
	fully human receptor antagonist
	can use with methotrexate

Infliximab (Remicade®)

Mechanism:	inhibits TNF-α (TM and soluble)
Excretion:	
Dosing:	3 mg/kg IV infusion q 8 weeks
	start 3 mg/kg IV $\times$ 1 on weeks 0, 2, 6 – may increase to 10 mg/kg or frequency to q 4 weeks
Pregnancy cat.:	**B**
Side effects:	infusion reactions; CNS disorders; hematologic abn; opportunistic infections
Monitoring:	WBC; baseline PPD
Notes:	FDA approval for Crohn's and rheumatoid arthritis
	not approved for pediatric use
	can use with methotrexate

Topical Corticosteroids

Group	Vehicle	Strength (%)
I (super-high potency)		
Betamethasone dipropionate	C, G, L, O	0.05
Clobetasol propionate	C, F, G, O, S Shampoo	0.05
Diflorasone diacetate	C, O	0.05
Halobetasol	C, O	0.05
II (high potency)		
Amcinonide	C, L, O	0.1
Betamethasone dipropionate	C, G, L, O	0.05
Desoximetasone	C	0.05, 0.25
	G	0.05
	O	0.25
Diflorasone	C, O	0.05
Fluocinonide	C, G, L, O	0.05
Halcinonide	C, O, S	0.1
Mometasone	C, L, O	0.1
III (potent)		
Amcinonide	C, L, O	0.1
Betamethasone dipropionate	C, L, O	0.05
	C, L, O	0.1
Desoximetasone	C	0.05, 0.25
	G	0.05
	O	0.25
Diflorasone	C, O	0.05
Fluocinonide	C	0.05

Group	Vehicle	Strength (%)
Fluticasone	O	0.005
	C	0.05
Halcinonide	C, O, S	0.1
Triamcinolone	C	.025, 0.1, 0.5
	O	0.1
	L	0.025, 0.1%
IV (mid potency)		
Betamethasone valerate	F	0.12
Clocortolone	C	0.1
Fluocinolone	C	0.01, 0.025
	O	0.025
	S	0.01
Flurandrenolide	C	0.025, 0.5
	O	0.05
	L	0.05
	Tape	
Hydrocortisone	C	2.5
Hydrocortisone valerate	C, O	0.2
Prednicarbate	C, O	0.1
Mometasone	C, L, O	0.1
Triamcinolone	C	.025, 0.1, 0.5
	O	0.1
	L	0.025, 0.1
	Paste	0.1
V (mid potency)		
Aclometasone	O	0.05
Betamethasone dipropionate	C, L, O	0.05
Betamethasone valerate	C, L, O	0.1

Group	Vehicle	Strength (%)
Desonide	C, L, O, S	0.05
Fluocinonide	Shampoo	0.01
Fluocinolone	C	0.01, 0.025
	O	0.025
	S	0.01
Flurandrenolide	C	0.025, 0.5
	O	0.05
	L	0.05
	Tape	
Fluticasone	O	0.005
	C	0.05
Hydrocortisone butyrate	C, O, S	0.1
Hydrocortisone valerate	C, O	0.2
Prednicarbate	C, O	0.1
Triamcinolone	C	.025, 0.1, 0.5
	O	0.1
	L	0.025, 0.1

VI (low potency)

Aclometasone	C, O	0.05
Betamethasone valerate	C, L, O	0.1
Desonide	C, L, O	0.05
Fluocinolone	C	0.01, 0.025
	O	0.025
	S	0.01
Triamcinolone	C	.025, 0.1, 0.5
	O	0.1
	L	0.025, 0.1

Group	Vehicle	Strength (%)
VII (low potency)		
Hydrocortisone	C, L, O, S	0.5, 1, 2.5
Hydrocortisone / urea	C	1 / 10
Hydrocortisone / pramoxine	C	1 / 1
	C, L, O	2.5 / 1

Key: F = foam, G = gel, O = ointment, C = cream, L = lotion, S = solution

Corticosteroid Potency

Short Acting	Equivalent Dose	GC[1] Potency	MC[2] Potency
Cortisone	25	0.8	2+
Hydrocortisone	20	1	2+
Intermediate			
Prednisone	5	4	1+
Prednisolone	5	4	1+
Methylprednisolone	4	5	0
Triamcinolone	4	5	0
Long-Acting			
Dexamethasone	0.75	20–30	0
Betamethasone	0.6–0.75	20–30	0

[1] *Glucocorticoid effects*:
- gluconeogenesis
- peripheral insulin resistance (hyperglycemia)
- ↑hepatic glycogen storage
- lipolysis (hypertriglyceridemia; fat redistribution)

[2] *Mineralococorticoid effects*:
- Na^+ reabsorption
- K^+ excretion → hypokalemia

Caution risk of avascular necrosis with any systemic steroid!!

Antihistamines

Drug	Mech[1]	Met/Excr	Dose	Pregnancy
Diphenhydramine (Benadryl)	H1 (ns)	hepatic/urine	25–50 mg q6–8°	B
Promethazine (Phenergan)	H1 (ns)	hepatic/urine	12.5–25 mg q6–8°	C
Hydroxyzine (Atarax/Vistaril)	H1 (ns)	hepatic/urine	12.5–25 mg q6–8°	C
Doxepin (Sinequan)	H1 (ns)	hepatic/urine	10–75 mg qhs	C
Loratidine (Claritin)	H1 (s)	hepatic	10 mg qd	B
Desloratadine (Clarinex)	H1 (s)	hepatic/urine	5 mg po qd	C
Cetirizine (Zyrtec)	H1 (s)	min metab	10 mg qd	B
Fexofenadine (Allegra)	H1 (s)	not hepatic	180 mg qd	C

[1] ns = nonspecific; s = specific

side effects: sedation, hyperexcitability in children, impaired cognitive function, ↑appetite, GI effects, dysuria, erectile dysfunction, tachycardia, dysrhythmias, blurred vision

Hormone Antagonists

Spironolactone

Mechanism:	weak antiandrogen
Metabolism:	hepatic
Excretion:	hepatobiliary
Dosing:	Start 25–50 mg po qd
	Possible increase to 100–200 mg po qd
Pregnancy cat.:	**X**
Side effects:	hyperkalemia, gynecomastia, menstrual irregularities GI effects; weakness; muscle cramps
Monitoring:	K^+, blood pressure, weight
Notes:	2nd line use for refractory acne treatment

Finasteride

Mechanism:	androgen inhibitor (type II 5α-reductase inhibitor)
Metabolism:	hepatic
Excretion:	urine and feces
Dosing:	1 mg po qd
Pregnancy cat.:	**X**
Side effects:	uncommon cases of sexual dysfunction
Monitoring:	none
Notes:	lack of proven efficacy in female pattern alopecia

Sawaya M. Antiandrogens and androgen inhibitors. In: Wolverton SE, ed. Comprehensive Dermatologic Drug Therapy. Philadelphia: W. B. Saunders Co. 2001: pp. 385–401.

Miscellaneous Drugs

Colchicine

Mechanism:	prevents assembly of tubule subunits into microtubules
Metabolism:	hepatic
Excretion:	bile and feces
Dosing:	0.6 mg po bid – tid
Pregnancy cat.:	**C** (parenteral D)
Side effects:	GI effects (diarrhea)
Monitoring:	CBC, UA, LFT, chemistry panel q 3 months
Notes:	need to shield from UV light exposure

Ivermectin

Mechanism:	blocks glutamate-gated Cl channels
Metabolism:	hepatic
Excretion:	feces
Dosing:	200 mg/kg $\times$ 1 dose (may repeat in 1 week) for scabies
Pregnancy cat.:	**C**
Side effects:	few
Monitoring:	none
Notes:	supplied in 6 mg tablets
	useful in recalcitrant/persistent scabies infestations

Nicotinamide

Mechanism:	suppression of antigen/mitogen-induced lymphoblast transformation
Metabolism:	
Excretion:	
Dosing:	200–500 mg po tid

Pregnancy cat.:	**C**
Side effects:	headache, GI effects
Monitoring.:	none
Notes:	niacin deficiency causes pellagra

Permethrin (Elimite)

Mechanism:	disrupts Na^+ transport
Metabolism:	hepatic
Excretion:	urine
Dosing:	apply 5% cream below neck for 8–14 hours
Pregnancy cat.:	**B**
Side effects:	burning, pruritus
Monitoring:	none
Notes:	avoid with allergy to formaldehyde

Saturated Solution of Potassium Iodide (SSKI)

Mechanism:	alters host immune/non-immune response
Metabolism:	none
Excretion:	urine
Dosing:	5 drops tid (may gradually titrate to 10 drops tid)
Pregnancy cat.:	**D**
Side effects:	rare (hypothyroidism)
Monitoring:	thyroid profile
Notes:	monitor for Wolff-Chaikoff effect

Thalidomide

Mechanism:	hypnosedative effects, immunomodulatory/anti-inflammatory effects (TNF-α), neural/vascular effects
Metabolism:	hepatic
Excretion:	nonrenal
Dosing:	50–200 mg/day (for lupus erythematosus)
Pregnancy cat.:	X
Side effects:	sedation
	teratogen
	peripheral sensory neuropathy
Monitoring:	CBC, β-HCG, LFTs
	Assess for sensory neuropathy (SNAP amplitude)
Notes:	STEPS program for pregnancy prevention

Davis L. Newer uses of older drugs – An update. In: Wolverton SE, ed. Comprehensive Dermatologic Drug Therapy. Philadelphia: W. B. Saunders Co. 2001: pp. 426–444.

PUVA Therapy

Methoxysoralen (8-methoxypsoralen) (Oxsoralen Ultra)

Mechanism:	selective immunosuppression at cutaneous level
Metabolism:	hepatic
Excretion:	urine and feces ($\leq$12 hours)
Dosing:	0.4 mg/kg 1–2 hrs. prior to UVA radiation
Pregnancy cat.:	**C**
Side effects:	nausea, erythema, pruritus
Notes:	UVA: 320–400 nm
	food intake slows absorption and
	$\downarrow$ peak blood level
	use protective eyewear for 24 hours

kg	Dose
<30	10 mg
3–65	20 mg
6–90	30 mg
>90	40 mg

Skin Types

I	always burns, never tans	white
II	always burns, sometimes tans	white
III	sometimes burns, always tans	white
IV	rarely burns, always tans	olive
V	never burns; always tans	brown skin
VI	never burns; tans darkly	black skin

UVA and UVB based on skin types

	UVA			UVB	
Skin type	Initial dose (J/cm^2)	Increment	Max	Initial dose (mJ/cm^2)	Increment
I	0.5–1.0	0.25–.5	5	5–10	5–10
II	1.0–2.0	0.25–.5	8	10–20	10–20
III	2.0–3.0	0.25–.5	12	20–30	20–30
IV	3.0–4.0	0.5–1	14	30–40	30–40
V	4.0–5.0	0.5–1	16	40–50	40–50
VI	5.0–6.0	0.5–1	20	50–70	50–60

Notes:

- treat patient with atopic dermatitis or erythroderma as type 1
- for symptomatic erythema (resolved), ↓ dose by 10%
- for symptomatic erythema (persistent), stop treatment until resolved, then resume at 25% lower dose

Morison WL. PUVA Photochemotherapy. In: Wolverton SE, ed. Comprehensive Dermatologic Drug Therapy. Philadelphia: W. B. Saunders Co. 2001: pp. 311–325.

Bowman PH. MCG Phototherapy Manual 1999.

Dermatology Pearls

Steroidogenesis

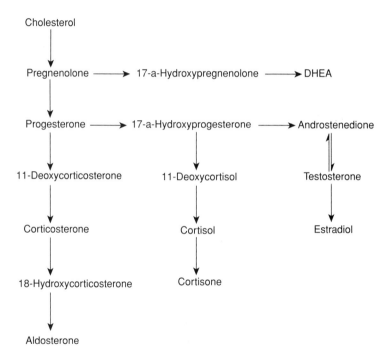

Collagen

Type	Chromosome	Tissue Distribution	Disease
I	17q21.3–22	Skin, bone, tendon	Ehlers-Danlos syndrome Osteogenesis imperfecta
II	7q21.3–q22	Cartilage, vitreous	Relapsing polychondritis
III	12q13–q14	Fetal skin, BV, GI tract	Ehlers-Danlos syndrome
IV	13q34, 2q, Xq22	BM (ubiquitous)	Alport syndrome, Goodpasture's syndrome
V	9q34.2–q34.3	Ubiquitous	Ehlers–Danlos syndrome
VI	21q22.3, 2q37	Aortic intima, placenta	
VII	3p21	Amnion, anchoring fibrils	Epidermolysis bullosa (EB), dystrophic EB, bullous lupus
VIII	3q, 1p	Endothelial cells	
IX	6q12–q14, 1p32	Cartilage	
X	6q12–q14, 1p32	Cartilage	
XI	1p21	Cartilage	

Type	Chromosome	Tissue Distribution	Disease
XII	6	Tendons, ligaments, perichondrium, periosteum	
XIII	10q22	Ubiquitous	
XIV	8q23	Skin, tendons, cornia	
XV	9q21–22	Ubiquitous	
XVI	1p34–35	Ubiquitous	
XVII	10q24.3	Hemidesmo somes	Bullous pemphigoid Herpes gestationis
XVIII	21q22.3	Ubiquitous Basement membrane	
XIX	6q12–q14, 1p32	Ubiquitious Basement membrane	
XX	6p12–q13		
XXI	6p11–12		

Uitto J et al. Collagen. In: Freedberg IM et al., eds. Fitzpatrick's Dermatology in General Medicine, 6 ed. New York, NY: McGraw-Hill 2003: pp. 167–168.

Keratins

Type II	Type I	Location
1	10	Suprabasal keratinocytes
1	9	Palmoplantar suprabasal keratinocytes
2e	10	Granular layer of epidermis
3	12	Cornea
4	13	Mucosal epithelium
5	14	Basal keratinocytes
5	15	Basal layer of nonkeratinizing epithelia
6a	16	Outer root sheath, hyperproliferative keratinocytes, palmoplantar
6b	17	Nail bed, epidermal appendages
7		Various patterns in transformed cells
8	18	Simple epithelia
	19	Embryonic
	20	Merkle cells
	21	Intestinal epithelia

Keratins in Disease

Keratin	Disease
1	Nonepidermolytic palmoplantar keratoderma
1, 10	Epidermolytic hyperkeratosis
2e	Ichthyosis bullosa of Siemens
3, 12	Corneal dystrophy of Meesmann
4, 13	White sponge nevus of Canon
5, 14	Epidermolysis bullosa simplex
6a, 16	Pachyonychia congenita, Jadassohn-Lewandowsky (type 1)

Keratin	*Disease*
9	Epidermolytic palmoplantar keratoderma
16	Focal nonepidermolytic palmoplantar keratoderma
17	Pachyonchia congenita, Jackson-Lawler (type 2)

Kimyai-Asadi A et al. Epidermal cell kinetic, epidermal differentiation, and keratinization. In: Freedberg IM et al., eds. Fitzpatrick's Dermatology in General Medicine, 6th ed. New York, 2003, p. 90–91.

Antigens in Dermatologic Diseases

Antigen	Size (kD)	Disease
Anti-epiligrin (laminin V)		Cicatricial pemphigoid
		Junctional EB (Herlitz)
BPAg1	230	Bullous pemphigoid
		Paraneoplastic pemphigus
BPAg2 (type XVII collagen)	180	Herpes gestationis
		Bullous pemphigoid
		Cicatricial pemphigoid
Desmocollin I		IgA pemphigus
		Subcorneal pustular dermatosis
Desmocollin II		
Desmoglein 1	160	Pemphigus foliaceous
Desmoglein 3	130	Pemphigus vulgaris, paraneoplastic pemphigus
Desmoplakin I	250	Paraneoplastic pemphigus
Desmoplakin II	210	Paraneoplastic pemphigus
Envoplakin	210	Paraneoplastic pemphigus
Periplakin	190	Paraneoplastic pemphigus
Type VII collagen	190	Bullous lupus erythematosus
Plakoglobin	85	Naxos disease

Antigen	Size (kD)	Disease
Plectin	580	EB simplex (with muscular dystrophy); paraneoplastic pemphigus
	97	Linear IgA disease

Antigens in Paraneoplastic pemphigus

Plectin	580 kD
BP 230	230 kD
Desmoplakin I	250 kD
Desmoplakin II	210 kD
Envoplakin	210 kD
Periplakin	190 kD
Unknown Ag	170 kD
Desmoglein 3	130 kD

Histochemical Staining

Stain	Purpose
Hematoxylin-Eosin	Routine
Masson trichome	Collagen
Verhoeff-von Gieson	Elastic fibers
Pinkus acid orcein	Elastic fibers
Silver nitrate	Melanin, reticulum fibers
Fontana-Masson	Melanin
Methenamine silver	Fungi, Donovan bodies, Frisch bacilli, basement membrane
Grocott	Fungi
Periodic acid-Schiff (PAS)	Glycogen, neutral MPS, fungi
Alcian blue, pH 2.5	Acid MPS
Alcian blue, pH 0.5	Sulfated MPS
Toluidine blue	Acid MPS
Colloidal iron	Acid MPS
Hyaluronidase	Hyaluronic acid
Mucicarmine	"Epithelial" mucin
Giemsa	Mast cell granules, acid MPS, myeloid granules, *Leishmania*
Fite	Acid-fast bacilli
Perls pottasium ferrocyanide	Hemosiderin
Alkaline Congo red	Amyloid
Von Kossa	Calcium
Scarlet red	Lipids
Oil red O	Lipids

Dopa (unfixed tissue)	Tyrosinase
Warthin-Starry	Spirochetes
Stain	**Purpose**
Dieterle and Steiner	Spirochetes, bacillary angiomatosis

Elenitsas R et al. Laboratory methods. In: Elder D, ed. Lever's Histopathology of the Skin. Lippincott-Raven, New York. 1997: p. 53.

Immunohistochemical Staining

Epidermal   (Cytokeratins – epithelial neoplasms)
  Cytokeratin 20   Merkel cell carcinoma
  Cytokeratin 7   Paget's disease
  EMA   Eccrine, apocrine, sebaceous glands
  CEA   Metastatic adenocarcinoma,
                      extramammary Paget's,
                      eccrine/apocrine gland

Mesenchymal
  Desmin   Muscle (all 3 types)
  Vimentin   Cells of mesenchymal origin
  Actin   Muscle
  CD31   Endothelial tumors: angiosarcoma
  CD34   DFSP: CD34+, XIIIa – (DF: CD34–,
                      XIIIa+, ST3+)

Neuroectodermal
  S100   Melanocytes, nerve, Langerhans, eccrine,
                      apocrine, Chondrocytes (desmoplastic
                      melanoma S100 –)
  HMB-45   Premelanosome vesicles, melanocytic nevi
                      and MM (desmoplastic melanoma
                      HMB-45 –)
  MART-1   Melanocytic nevi and malignant melanoma

Hematopoietic
  CD45 (LAC)   CD45RO: memory T-cell; CD45RA: B cells,
                      naive T-cell
  CD20   Pan B-cell marker
  CD43 (Leu-22)   Pan T-cell marker

κ and λ	Mature B cells and plasma cells
CD30 (Ki-1)	Stains activated T and B cells, Reed–Sternberg cells, large cell, anaplastic CTCL, Lymphomatoid papulosis type A
CD68 (Kp-1)	Marker for histiocytes
Factor XIIIa	PLTs, macrophages, megakaryocytes, dendrites

Miscellaneous

BCL2	Follicular center lymphoma (B origin), BCC (bcl2 +)
CD1A (Leu-6)	Langerhans cells
CD3	Pan T-cell marker
CD4	T helper cells
CD8	T cytotoxic suppressor cells
CD20	Pan B-cell marker
CD31	Endothelial cell marker
CD34	Endothelial cells, dermal spindle cells
CD56	NK cells and angiocentric T-cell lymphoma
CD68	Histiocytes

Septal Panniculitides

With vasculitis

Small vessels

  Venules → LCV

Large vessels

  Veins → Superficial thrombophlebitis

  Arteries → Cutaneous polyarteritis nodosa

No vasculitis

Lymphocytes and plasma cells

  Granulomatous infiltrate in septa → Necrobiosis lipoidica

  No granulomatous infiltrate in septa → Scleroderma

Histiocytes mostly

  Granulomatous infiltrate

  Mucin in center of palisaded granulomas → Subcutaneous
    GA

  Fibrin in center of palisaded granulomas → Rheumatoid
    nodule

  Degenerated collagen, foamy histiocytes →
    Xanthogranuloma cholesterol clefts

  No mucin, fibrin, or degeneration of collagen → Erythema
    nodosum but with radial granulomas in septa

Requena L, Yus ES. Panniculitis. Part I. Mostly septal panniculitis.
J Am Acad Dermatol 2001; 45: 163–183.

Lobular Panniculitides

With vasculitis

Small vessels

Venules → Erythema nodosum leprosum, Lucio's phenomenon, Neutrophilic lobular (pustular) panniculitis with rheumatoid arthritis

Large vessels

Arteries → Erythema induratum of Bazin, Crohn's disease

No vasculitis

Few or no inflammatory cells

Necrosis at center of lobule → Sclerosing panniculitis

With vascular calcification → Calciphylaxis, Oxalosis

With needle-shaped crystals in adipocytes → Sclerema neonatorum

Lymphocytes predominate

Superficial and deep perivascular dermal infiltrate → Cold panniculitis

Lymphoid follicles, plasma cells and nuclear dust → Lupus panniculitis

Lymphocytes and plasma cells → Panniculitis in dermatomyositis

Neutrophils predominant

Fat necrosis with saponification of adipocytes → Pancreatic panniculitis

Neutrophils between collagen bundles of dermis → α1-antitrypsin deficiency

Bacteria, fungi, or protozoa (via special stains) → Infective panniculitis

Foreign bodies → Facticial panniculitis

No Vasculitis (continued)

Histiocytes predominant (granulomatous)

  No crystals in adipocytes → Subcutaneous sarcoidosis,
    Traumatic panniculitis, Lipoatrophy

  Crystals in histiocytes/adipocytes → Subcutaneous fat
    necrosis of newborn, Poststeroid panniculitis, Gout
    panniculitis

  Cytophagic histiocytes → Cytophagic histiocytic panniculitis

  Sclerosis of the septa → Postradiation
    pseudosclerodermatous panniculitis

Requena L, Yus ES. Panniculitis. Part II. Mostly lobular panniculitis. *J Am Acad Dermatol* 2001; 45: 325–361.

Dermatologic Signs

Albright's sign – dimple on 4th MCP (Gorlin's syndrome)

Asboe Hansen sign – extension of blister with direct pressure (pemphigus)

Auspitz sign – pinpoint bleeding upon scale removal (psoriasis)

Beighton's sign – thumb touches arm (EDS)

Berliner's sign – palpebral edema seen in exanthem subitum

Crowe's sign – axillary freckling (NF)

Darier's sign – whealing with skin striking (urticaria pigmentosa)

Deck-chair sign – skinfold sparing in papuloerythroderma of Ofuji

Dimple sign – dermatofibroma

Forscheimer's sign – enanthem on soft palate and uvula (Rubella)

Gorlin's sign – ability to touch tip of tongue to nose (Marfan syndrome)

Gottron's sign – eruption occurs on knuckles, knees and elbows (dermatomyositis)

Groove sign – eosinophilic fasciitis; lymphogranuloma venereum

Headlight sign – perinasal and periorbital pallor (atopic dermatitis)

Hertoghe's sign – thinning of the lateral eyebrows (atopic dermatitis)

Higoumènaki's sign – unilateral thickening of inner $\frac{1}{3}$ of clavicle (syphilis)

Hutchinson's sign – nasal tip zoster; warns of ophthalmic involvement with nasociliary branch

Hutchinson's sign: pigmentation over nail fold as indicator of melanoma

Nikolsky sign – extension of blister with lateral pressure (toxic epidermal necrolysis, pemphigus vulgaris, staphylococcal scalded skin syndrome, acute generalized exanthematous pustulosis)

Ollendorf's sign – exquisitely tender papule to blunt probe (2° syphilis)

Osler's sign – pigmentation of sclerae (alkaptonuria)

Rumpel-Leede sign – distal shower of petechiae that occurs immediately after release of pressure from tourniquet or sphygmomanometer

Russel's sign – excoriations on knuckles from anorexia

Shoulder pad sign – prominent deltoid muscle (1° systemic amyloidosis)

Sign of Leser-Trelat – sudden occurrence of seborrheic keratoses with underlying malignancy

Tent sign – pilomatricoma

Trousseau's sign – migratory thrombophlebitis with underlying malignancy

Winterbottom's sign – posterior cervical lymphadenopathy (African trypanosomiasis)

Leishmaniasis

Cutaneous leishmaniasis

Old World	*L. tropica*	Near East, USSR
(Phlebotomus)	*L. infantum*	Mediterranean rim
	L. major	Near East, Africa
	L. aethiopica	Ethiopia, Kenya
New World	*L. mexicana*	Mexico, C. America
(Lutzomyia)	*L. braziliensis*	Brazil, Bolivia
	L. amazonesis	Brazil

Mucocutaneous leishmaniasis

L. braziliensis
L. panamensis
L. amazonensis

Diffuse cutaneous leishmaniasis

| Old World | *L. aethiopica* | Ethiopia, Kenya |
| New World | *L. mexicana* | South America |

Visceral leishmaniasis

L. donovani   India, Kenya
L. infantum   Mediterranean rim

Uncommon forms of leishmaniasis

| L recidivans | *L. tropica* | Middle East, USSR |
| Post-kala-azar | *L. donovani* | India, Nepal, China |

Diseases and Etiology

Actinomyces	*Actinomyces israelii*
Amebiasis	*Entamoeba histolytica*
Anthrax	*Bacillus anthracis*
Aspergillosis	*Aspergillus flavus* (cutaneous); *Aspergillus fumigatus* (disseminated)
Bacillary angiomatosis	*Bartonella henselae* (vector: cat flea) *Bartonella quintana* (vector: body louse)
Bartonellosis / Carrion's disease	*B. bacilliformis* (vector: phlebotomus)
Bedbugs (Cimicidae)	*Cimex, Leptocimex, Oeciacus*
Bejel (endemic syphilis)	*Treponema pallidum* (ssp. *endemicum*)
Black piedra	*Piedra hortai*
Blastomycosis	*Blastomyces dermatitidis*
Botryomycosis	*S. aureus* (*E. coli, Proteus, Pseudomonas*)
Bouteonneuse fever	*Rickettsia conorii* (vector: tick)
Brill–Zinsser disease	*R. prowazeckii* same as epidemic typhus
Brucellosis	*B. melitensis* (goat), *B. suis* (pig), *B. abortus* (cow), *B. canis* (dog)
Bullous impetigo	*S. aureus* phage II grp 71 exfoliatin toxin
Buruli ulcer	*Mycobacterium ulcerans*
Carbuncle	*Staphylococcus aureus*

Caterpillar dermatitis	Gypsy moth, *Lymantria dispar*; Corn emperor moth, *Automeris io*; Puss caterpillar, *Megalopyge opercularis*
Cat-scratch disease	*Bartonella henselae* (vector: cat flea)
Cellulitis	*S. pyogenes, S. aureus, H. influenza* (children), *V. vulnificans*
Chagas disease	*Trypanosoma cruzi* (vector: triatomine)
Chancroid	*Hemophilus ducreyi*
Chickenpox	Varicella zoster virus
Chromoblastomycosis	*Cladosporium carrionii*
	Fonsecaea compacta
	Fonsecaea pedrosoi
	Phialophora verrucosae
	Rhinocladiella aquaspersa
Coddidiomycosis	*Coccidiodes immitis*
Cryptococcosis	*Cryptococcus neoformans*
Cutaneous larvae migrans	*Ancylostoma braziliense*
Cutaneous larvae currens	*Strongyloides stercoralis*
Cysticercosis	*Taenia solium* (pork tapeworm)
Dengue fever	*Flavivirus* (vector: *Aedes aegypti*)
Diptheria	*Corynebacterium diphtheriae*
Distal subungual onychomycosis	*Trichophyton rubrum*
Dracunculosis	*Dracunculus medinensis* (vector: Cyclops)

Ecthyma	Group A β-hemolytic strep (*S. pyogenes*), *S. aureus*
Ecthyma contagiosum (Orf)	Parapoxvirus
Ecthyma gangrenosum	*Pseudomonas aeruginosa*
Ehrlichiosis	*Ehrlichia chaffeensis*
Erysipelas	Group A β-hemolytic strep (*S. pyogenes*)
Erysipeloid	*Erysipelothrix rhusiopathiae*
Erythema chronicum migrans	*B. burgdorferi* (Lyme disease; *Ixodes*)
Erythema infectiosum (5th disease)	Parvovirus B-19
Erythrasma	*Corynebacterium minutissimum*
Exanthem subitum	Human herpesvirus 6 (HHV-6)
Filariasis	Brugia malayi-SE Asia/B. timor-Indonesia (vector: mosquito/Culex species)
Filariasis	*Wuchereria bancrofti* (Africa, Asia, Latin America) (vector: *Culex* mosquito)
Fire ant sting	*Solenopsis richteri* (black fire ant) *Solenopsis invicta* (red fire ant)
Fishtank granuloma	*Mycobacterium marinum*
Folliculitis	Mixed normal cutaneous flora
Furuncle	*S. aureus*
Fournier's gangrene	Group A Streptococcus (mixed infection)
Gianotti-Crosti syndrome	HBV, EBV, coxsackie enterovirus
Gonococcemia	*Neisseria gonorrheae*

Gram negative folliculitus	*Enterobacter, Klebsiella, Proteus*
Granuloma inguinale	*Calymmatobacterium granulomatis*
Hairly leukoplakia	EBV
Hand-foot-mouth disease	Coxsackie virus A 16
Herpangina	Coxsackie virus A 1–10
Histoplasmosis	*H. capsulatum; H. duboisii* (African)
Hot tub folliculitis	*Pseudomonas*
Impetigo contagiosum	Group A *Streptococcus*
Impetigo of Bockhart	*S. aureus*
Infectious mononucleosis	EBV, CMV
Kaposi's sarcoma	HHV-8
Leishmaniasis, localized	Old world: *L. major* New world: *L braziliensis, L. mexicana*
Leishmaniasis, diffuse	Old world: *L. aethiopica* New world: *L amazonensis*
Leishmaniasis, recidivans	Old world: *L. tropica* New world: *L. braziliensis*
Leishmaniasis, post kala-azar	Old world: *L. donovani* New world: *L. tropica*
Leishmaniasis, mucocutaneous	New world: *L. braziliensis, panamensis*
Leishmaniasis, visceral (kala-azar)	Old world: *L. donovani, L. tropica* New world: *L. donovani chagasi*
Leishmaniasis, vectors	Old world: Phlebotomus New world: Lutzomyia
Leprosy	*Mycobacterium leprae*

Leptospirosis	Pretibial fever (anicteric leptospirosis: *Leptospira autumnalis*)
	Weil's disease (icteric leptospirosis: *L. interrogans*)
Loiasis	Loa loa (vector: deer fly, *Chrysops*)
Lyme disease	*B. burgdorferi* (vector-deer tick, *I. scapularis/dammini* in NE and MW U.S., *I. pacificus* in NW, *I. ricinus* in Europe)
Lymphogranuloma venereum	*Chlamydia trachomatis*
Malakoplakia	*E. coli, S. aureus*
Malaria	*Plasmodium* species (vector: *Anopheles*)
Measles (rubeola)	Paramyxovirus
Milker's nodule	Parapoxvirus
Molluscum contagiosum	Poxvirus
Moth dermatitis (Lepidopterism)	Hylesia moth venom
Mycetoma (Madura foot)	
Eumycetoma	*Pseudallescheria boydii, Madurella mycetomi, M. grisea, Phialophora jeanselmei*
Actinomycetoma	*N. brasiliensis, N. asteroides, N. madurae, Streptomyces pelletieri, S. somaliensis, A. israelii*
Myiasis	
Furuncular	*Dermatobia hominis* (human botfly)
Accidental/wound	*Musca domestica* (common housefly)

Necrotizing fasciitis, type I	Bowel-associated infection (*Enterobacter, Enterococcci, B. fragilis*)
Necrotizing fasciitis, type II	*S. pyogenes, Vibrio vulnificans* (rare)
Nocardiosis	*Nocardia asteroides*
Onchocerciasis	*Onchocerca volvulus* (vector: black fly)
Orf	Parapoxvirus
Paracoccidiomycosis	*Paracoccidiodes brasiliensis*
Paronychia	Candida, gram (–) bacteria, *Staph, Strep*
Pediculosis capitis	*Pediculus humanus capitis*
Pediculosis corporis	*Pediculus humanus corporis*
Pediculosis pubis	*Phthirus pubis*
Pinta	*Treponema carateum*
Pinworm (enterobiasis)	*Enterobius vermicularis*
Pitted keratolysis	*C. minutissimum*
	Dermatophilus congolensis
	Micrococcus sedentarius
Plague, bubonic	*Yersinia pestis* (vector: rat flea)
	Xenopsylla cheopsis, Pulex irritans
Psittacosis	*Chlamydia psittaci*
Purpura fulminans	Group A Streptococcus
Pyomyositis	*S. aureus*
Q fever	*Rickettsia/Coxiella burnetti*
Queensland tick typhus	*Rickettsia australis* (vector: tick, Ixodes)

Reiter's syndrome	*Chlamydia, Shigella, Salmonella, Yersinia, Campyloacter, Ureaplasma, Mycoplasma, B. burgdorferi*
Relapsing fever (tick fever)	*Borrelia recurrentis, B. duttonii* (vector: tick)
Rift valley fever	Phlebovirus-bunyavirus family (*Aedes*)
Rhinoscleroma	*Klebsiella rhinoscleromatis*
Rhinosporidiosis	*Rhinosporidium seeberi*
Rickettsialpox	*Rickettsia akari* (vector: mouse mite *Liponyssoides sanguineus*)
Rocky mountain spotted fever	*R. rickettsii* (vector: *D. andersoni* in west; *D. variabilis* in southeast)
Roseola infantum	HHV-6
Rubella	Togavirus
Scabies	*Sarcoptes scabiei var. hominis*
Scarlet fever	Group A Streptococcus
Schistosomiasis	*S. haematobium, S. mansoni, S. japonicum*
Seabather's eruption (salt)	Sea anemone, *Edwardsiella lineata* Thimble jellyfish, *Linuche unguiculata*
Seaweed dermatitis (salt)	Toxins from blue-green algae, *Lyngya ma*
Smallpox	Variola (orthopox virus)
South American blastomycosis	*Paracoccidiodes brasiliensis*
Black widow	*Lactrodectus mactans*
Brown recluse	*Loxosceles reclusa*

Sporotrichosis	*Sporothrix schenckii*
Strongyloidiasis	*Larva currens* (*Strongyloides stercoralis*)
Staph scalded skin syndrome	*S. aureus* phage II, group 71 and 55
Swimmer's itch (fresh, salt)	Schistosome cercariae
Syphilis	*Treponema pallidum*
Tinea barbae	*T. cerrucosum, T. mentagrophyte*
Tinea capitis	*T. tonsurans* (anthropophilic, U.S.)
	M. canis (zoophilic, Europe)
	T. violaceum (Africa)
	M. ferrugineum (SE Asia)
Tinea corporis	*T. rubrum* (anthropophilic)
	M. canis (zoophilic)
	M. gypseum (geophilic)
Tinea cruris	*T. rubrum, E. floccosum*
Tinea facei	*T. rubrum, T. tonsurans*
Tinea imbricata	*T. concentricum*
Tinea nigra	*Phaeoannellomyces werneckii*
Tinea pedis/manum	*T. rubrum/mentagrophytes, E. floccosum*
Tinea versicolor	*Malassezia furfur*
Tinea unguium	*T. rubrum*
Toxoplasmosis	*Toxoplasmosis canii*
Trichinosis	*Trichinella spiralis*
Trichomycosis axillaris	*Corynebacterium tenuis*
Trypanosomiasis, African	*Trypanosma brucei gambiense* (west) *Trypanosoma brucei rhodesiense* (east)

Trypanosomiasis, American	*Trypanosoma cruzi*
Tuberculosis	*Mycobacterium tuberuculosis*
Tularemia	*Francisella tularensis* (*D. andersoni, D. variabilis, I. ricinus*)
Tungiasis	Burrowing flea, *Tunga penetrans*
Typhus, Endemic	*Rickettsia typhi* (rat flea feces, *Xenopsylla cheopis, X. braziliensis*)
Typhus, Epidemic	*Rickettsia prowazeckii* (body louse feces, *Pediculus* species)
Typhus, Scrub	*Rickettsia tsutsugamushi* (red chigger)
Vaccinia	Orthopox virus

Verruca associations

Actinic keratosis	HPV-36
Bowen's disease	HPV-34
Bowenoid papulosis	HPV-16, 18, 33, 34, 42
Butcher's warts	HPV-7
Cervical cancer	HPV-16, 18, 31, 33, 35, 39
Condyloma acuminate	HPV-6, 11, 16, 18
Condyloma, flat	HPV-42
Epidermodysplasia verruciformis	HPV-5, 8, 9 10, 12, 14, 15, 17, 19–29
Focal epithelial hyperplasia	HPV-13, 32
Genital papilloma	HPV-42
Keratoacanthoma	HPV-36, 37
Malignant melanoma	HPV-38
Laryngeal papilloma	HPV-6, 11
Laryngeal carcinoma	HPV-30, 40

Verruca, palatal	HPV-2
Verruca, plana	HPV-3, 10, 41
Verruca, vulgaris	HPV-2, 7
Verruca, filiform	HPV-2
Weil's disease	*see* Leptospirosis
White piedra	*Trichosporon beigelii*
White superficial onychomycosis	*Trichophyton mentagrophytes, T. rubrum*
Woolsorter's disease	Anthrax (*B. anthracis*)
Yaws	*Treponema pallidum* (spp *pertenue*)
Yellow fever	Yellow fever virus (vector: *Aedes aegypti*)

Autosomal Dominant Diseases

Disease	Gene
Bannayan–Riley–Ruvalcaba	PTEN
Bart's syndrome	COL7A1 – type VII collagen
Bullous ichthyosiform erythroderma	Keratins 1 and 10
Bullous Ichhtyosis of Siemens	Keratin 2e
Carney complex (LAMB, NAME)	PRKAR1A
Citrullinemia	Arginosuccinate synthetase
Cowden's syndrome	PTEN
Darier–White disease	SERCA2 – Ca ATPase 2A2
Dominant dystrophic EB	COL7A1 – type VII collagen
Dyskeratosis congenita	TERC – telomerase
EBS	Keratins 5 and 14
Ectodermal dysplasia/skin fragility	Plakophilin 1
Erythrokeratoderma variabilis	Connexin 31
Gardner's syndrome	APC
Gorlin's syndrome	PTCH
Hailey–Hailey disease	ATPase 2C1
Hereditary angioedema (Quinke's)	C1 INH – C1 esterase inihibitor
Hereditary Hemorrhagic Telang	Endoglein
Hidrotic ED (Clouston's)	Connexin 30
MEN I	MEN I – menin
MEN IIa and IIb	RET – receptor tyrosine kinase
Milroy's disease	FLT-4

Disease	Gene
Monilethrix	KRT hHb6 and hHb1 type II
Muir–Torre syndrome	hMSH2
Nail–patella syndrome	LMX1B
Naxos disease	Junctional plakoglobin
Neurofibromatosis I	NF-1 – neurofibromin
Neurofibromatosis II	NF-2 – Schwannomin/Merlin
Peutz-Jeghers syndrome	STK11
Piebaldism	C-kit
Porphyria cutanea tarda	Uroporphyrinogen decarboxylase
Porphyria, acute intermittent	Porphobilinogen deaminase
Porphyria, hereditary coproporphyria	Coproporphyrinogen oxidase
Porphyria, variegate	Protoporphyrinogen oxidase
Rubenstein–Taybi syndrome	CBP – CREB binding protein
Striate PPK 1	Desmoglein-1
Striate PPK 2	Desmoplakin
Tuberous sclerosis	TSC1 (9 – hamartin)
Tuberous sclerosis	TSC2 (16 – tuberin)
Vohwinkel's	Loricrin
Vohwinkel's with deafness	Connexin 26
Vorner's syndrome	Keratin 9
Waardenburg's syndrome	PAX3
White sponge nevus	Keratin 4 and 13

Autosomal Recessive Diseases

Disease	Gene
Alkaptonuria	Homogentisic acid oxidase
Ataxia–telangiectasia (Louis-Barr)	ATM
Atrichia with papules	HR – hairless gene
Bloom's syndrome	BLM; RECQL3
Chediak–Higashi syndrome	LYST
Cockayne's syndrome	CKN1; ERCC6 – CPB DNA helicase
Conradi–Hunermann syndrome	PEX7
EBS with Myotonic dystrophy	Plectin
Gaucher's disease	Beta-glucocerebrosidase
Griscelli syndrome	MTO5a – myosin-Va
Homocystinuria	Cystathione synthetase
Hurler's syndrome	Alpha-L-uronidase
Ichthyosis, Lamellar	Transglutaminase-1
Junctional EB (EB letalis, Hurlitz)	Laminin 5
Junctional EB with pyloric atresia	Integrin (alpha 6, beta 4)
Niemann–Pick disease	Sphyingomyelinase
Netherton's syndrome	SPINK5
Oculocutaneous albinism I	tyrosinase
Oculocutaneous albinism II	P gene
Oculocutaneous albinism III	TRP1 – tyrosine related protein
Papillon–Lefevre syndrome	Cathepsin C
Phenylketonuria	Phenylalanine hydroxylase
PIBIDS	TFIIH
Porphyria, congenital erythropoietic	Urophorphyrinogen III cosynthase

Disease	Gene
Refsum syndrome	Phytanoyl Co-A hydroxylase
Richner–Hanhart syndrome	Tyrosinase aminotransferase
Rothmund–Thompson syndrome	RECQL4
SCID	adenosine deaminase IL-2 receptor (10 + gene defects)
Sjogren–Larsson syndrome	Fatty aldehyde dehydrogenase
Takahara's disease	Catalase
Tangier disease	CERP
Werner's syndrome	WRN; ERCDC
Xeroderma pigmentosa	DNA helicase

X-Linked Dominant Diseases

Disease	Gene
CHILD syndrome	EBP – emopamil binding protein
Conradi–Hunermann syndrome	EPP
Incontinentia pigmenti	NEMO
Goltz syndrome	

X-Linked Recessive Diseases

Disease	Gene
Bruton's agammaglobulinemia	BTK
Chronic granulomatous disease	Cytochrome b
Cutis laxa	Fibulin/elastin
Dyskeratosis congenita	Dyskerin
Fabry's disease	Alpha-galactosidase A
Hunter's syndrome	Iduronate sulfatase
Anhidrotic ectodermal dysplasia	Ectodysplasin
Ichthyosis, X-linked	Aryl sulfatase C
Lesch–Nyhan syndrome	HGPRT
Menke's kinky hair syndrome	MNKSCID
Wiskott–Aldrich syndrome	WASP

Syndromes

Achenbach's syndrome	paroxysmal hand hematoma
Adams-Oliver syndrome	aplasia cutis congenita of scalp
	cutis marmorata
	telangiectasia congenita
	limb defects
AEC syndrome (Hay-Wells syndrome)	ankyloblepharon
	ectodermal defects
	cleft lip and/or palate
AHYS syndrome	acquired hyperostosis syndrome
Alagille's syndrome	intrahepatic bile ductular atresia
	patent extrahepatic bile ducts
	characteristic facies
	cardiac murmur
	vertebral and ocular
	abnormalities
	low intelligence
	hypogonadism
Alezzandrini's syndrome	unilateral degenerative retinitis
	subsequent ipsilateral vitiligo,
	poliosis
ANOTHER syndrome	alopecia
	nail dystrophy
	ophthalmic complications
	thyroid dysfunction
	hypohidrosis
	ephelides
	enteropathy
	respiratory tract infections

APECED syndrome	autoimmune polyendocrinopathy candidiasis ectodermal dystrophy
Apert's syndrome	synostosis of feet, hands carpi, tarsi, cervical vertebrae, skull
Ascher syndrome	progressive enlargement of upper lip blepharochalasis
Baboon syndrome	erythematous plaques on buttocks
Bannayan–Riley–Ruvalcaba syndrome	lipomas and vascular malformations lentigines of penis and vulva verrucae acanthosis nigricans
Bannworth's syndrome	focal, severe, radicular pains lymphocytic meningitis CN paralysis
Bare lymphocyte syndrome	defects in HLA class I expression
Barraquer–Simon's syndrome	progressive lipodystrophy
Bart's syndrome	dominant dermolytic epidermal bullosa
Bazex's syndrome	underlying malignancy neoplasm of aerodigestive tract; (acrokeratosis paraneoplastica)

Beals–Hecht syndrome	arachnodactyly
	narrow body habitus
	scoliosis
	congenital contractures
	external ear deformities
Beckwith–Wiedemann syndrome	facial port-wine stain
	macroglossia
	omphalocele
	visceral hyperplasia
	occasionally hemihypertrophy
	hypoglycemia
Beradinelli–Seip syndrome	congenital total lipodystrophy
BIDS syndrome	brittle hair
	impaired intelligence
	decreased fertility
	short stature
	(IBIDS: + ichthyosis
	PIBIDS: + photosensitivity)
Birt–Hogg–Dube syndrome	fibrofolliculomas
	acrochordons
	collagenomas, lipomas, fibromas
Bjornstad's syndrome	congenital cochlear deafness
	pili torti
Bloom syndrome	telangiectatic malar erythema
	photosensitivity
	facial telangiectasia
	short stature
	immunodeficiency
Blue rubber bleb nevus syndrome	cutaneous/GI venous malformations

Bluefarb–Stewart syndrome	reddish purple nodules/plaque
	resembles Kaposi's sarcoma
Brooke–Fordyce syndrome	cylindromas
	trichoepitheliomas
Brooke–Spiegler syndrome	cylindromas
	trichoepitheliomas
	spiradenomas
Caldwell's syndrome	acquired angioedema I
Cardio–Facio–Cutaneous Syndrome	craniofacial appearance
	psychomotor and growth retardation
	congenital cardiac defects
	skin and hair abnormalities
Cartilage–hair hypoplasia syndrome	short-limbed dwarfism
	fine, sparse, hypopigmented hair
	defective cell-mediated immunity
Chanarin–Dorfman syndrome	ichthyosiform eruption
	myopathy
	vacuolated leukocytes
Chediak–Higashi syndrome	oculocutaneous albinism
	immunologic deficiency
CHILD syndrome	congenital hemidysplasia
	ichthyosiform erythroderma
	limb defects
CHIME syndrome	colobomas of eye
	heart defects
	ichthyosiform dermatits
	mental retardation
	ear defects

Christ–Siemens–Touraine syndrome	hypotrichosis
	anodontia
	hypohidrosis / anhidrosis
Churg–Straus syndrome	asthma
	eosinophilia
	vasculitis
Clouston's syndrome	hidrotic ectodermal dysplasia
	alopecia
	nail dystrophy
	palmoplantar hyperkeratosis
	eye changes
Cobb syndrome	port-wine hemangioma / vascular
	malformation near dermatome
Cockayne's syndrome	syndrome of premature aging
	dwarfism
	retinal atrophy
	deafness
Cogan's syndrome	nonsyphilitic interstital keratitis (bilateral)
	vestibuloauditory symptoms
COIF syndrome	congenital onychodysplasia, index fingers
Comel–Netherton syndrome	ichthyosis linearis circumflexa
	trichorrhexis invaginata
	atopic diathesis
Conradi–Hünermann syndrome	chondrodysplasia punctata is variant

Cooks syndrome	bilateral nail hypoplasia of digits 1–3
	absence of nails of digits 4 and 5
	total absence of toenails
	absence of distal phalanges
Cornelia de Lange syndrome	hyptertrichosis
Costello syndrome	growth retardation
	coarse facies
	redundant skin (neck, hands, soles)
	dark skin / acanthosis nigricans
	nasal papillomata
Cowden's syndrome	multiple benign and malignant tumors
Crandall's syndrome	pili torti
	nerve deafness
	hypogonadism
Cronkhite–Canada syndrome	alopecia
	skin pigmentation
	onychodystrophy
	malabsorption
	generalized GI polyposis
	melanotic macules on fingers
Cross–McKusick–Breen syndrome	white skin
	blond hair/yellow-gray metallic
	cloudy corneas
	jerky nystagmus
	gingival fibromatosis
	retardation
Crow-Fukase syndrome	*see* POEMS syndrome

EEC syndrome	ectodermal dysplasia
	ectrodactyly
	cleft lip/palate
	lacks scalp dermatitis
Elejalde syndrome	pigment dilution
	silvery, metallic hair
	prominent neurologic defects
	no immune defects
Eosinophilia–myalgia syndrome	ingestion of L-tryptophan contaminated with 1, 1'-ethylidenebis
	similar to eosinophilic fasciitis
Epidermal nevus syndromes	Schimmelpenning syndrome
	nevus comedonicus
	pigmented hairy epidermal nevus
	Proteus syndrome
	CHILD syndrome
FACE syndrome	Facial Afro-Caribbean
	Childhood eruption (variant of granulomatous rosacea)
Favre–Racouchet syndrome	nodular elastoidosis
	cysts and comedones
Fish odor syndrome	excretion of trimethylamine
Frey syndrome	hyperemia of head and neck
	abundant gustatory sweating
	injury to of auriculotemporal nerve

Frohlich's syndrome   multiple lipomas
                                  obesity
                                  sexual infantism
Gardner's syndrome   intestinal polyposis and colon
                                      cancer
Gianotti–Crosti syndrome   papular acrodermatitis of
                                  childhood
Glucagonoma syndrome   necrolytic migratory erythema
                                  assoc. with pancreatic APUD
                                      tumor
Goltz syndrome   multiple abnormalities of
                                  mesodermal and ectodermal
                                  tissues
Good's syndrome   thymoma with
                                  immunodeficiency
Gorlin's (nevoid BCC)   multiple basal cell carcinomas
syndrome   odontogenic cysts of jaws
                                      palmar pits
                                  bone anomalies (ribs, spine,
                                      skull)
Gougerot–Blum syndrome   pigmented purpuric dermatosis
Graham Little syndrome   acuminate follicular papules
                                      alopecia
                                  lichen planus
Graham Little–Piccardi-   patchy cicatricila alopecia of
Lassueur   scalp
                                  follicular spinous papules of
                                      trunk, upper arms and legs,
                                  and scalp

Griscelli syndrome	variable pigmentary dilution
	silvery metallic hair
	frequent pyogenic infections
	neutropenia
	thrombocytopenia
Grönblad–Strandberg syndrome	angioid streaks with PXE
Hallermann–Streiff syndrome	birdlike facies with beaklike nose
	microphthalmia
	micrognathia
	congenital cataracts
	hypotrichosis
Happle syndrome	X-linked dominant chondrodysplasia punctata
Heerfordt's syndrome	uveoparotid fever
	parotid and lacrimal gland enlargement
	uveitis
	fever
	(may occur in sarcoidosis)
Hermansky–Pudlak syndrome	oculocutanous albinism
	hemorrhagic diathesis from absence of platelet dense bodies
	accumulation of ceroid-like material
Howel–Evan's syndrome	hereditary esophageal carcinoma
Hunter's syndrome	X-linked mucopolysaccharidosis

Hurler's syndrome	increased hair growth
	disorder of mucopolysaccharides
	deficiency of alpha-L-iduronidase
Hutchinson–Gilford syndrome (progeria)	dwarfism
	alopecia
	atrophy of skin and muscles
	large head and prominent scalp veins
	atherosclerosis
Hypereosinophila syndrome	eosinophilia >1500/mm^3 for >6 mo
Jadassohn–Lewandowsky syndrome	type 1 paronychia congenita
Jackson–Sertoli syndrome	type 2 paronychia congenita
Job's syndrome	hypergammaglobulinemia E
Kasabach–Merritt syndrome	consumptive coagulopathy (kaposiform hemangioendotheliomas)
KID syndrome	congenital ichthyosiform eruption
	neurosensory deafness hypotrichosis
	partial anhidrosis
	vascularity of cornea
	nail dystrophy
	tight heel cords

Kindler syndrome	blistering in infancy
	photosensitivity
	progressive poikiloderma
Klinefelter's syndrome	hypogonadism
	gynecomastia
	eunuchoidism
	small/absent testicles
	elevated gonadotropins
Klippel–Feil syndrome	low posterior scalp hairline
	extending onto shoulders
	short neck
	cervical vertebrae are fused
Klippel–Trenaunay syndrome	port-wine
	deep venous system
	malformation
	superficial varicosities
	bony and soft tissue
	hypertrophy
	(Parkes–Weber with AV fistula)
Kobberlin–Dunnigan syndrome	familial partial lipodystrophy
LAMB syndrome (NAME)	lentigines
	atrial myxoma
	mucocutaneous myxomas
	blue nevi
Laugier–Hunziker syndrome	pigmentation of the nails
	buccal and lip pigmentation
Ledderhose's syndrome	plantar fibromatosis (plantar
	analog of Dupuytren's
	contracture)

LEOPARD syndrome	Lentigines
	EKG abnormalities
	Ocular hypertelorism
	Pulmonary stenosis
	Abnormalities of genitalia
	Retardation of growth
	Mental deficiency
Lesch–Nyhan syndrome	childhood hyperuricemia
	choreoathetosis
	progressive mental retardation
	self-mutilation
	deficiency of HGPRT
Leser–Trélat syndrome	sudden onset of numerous
	seborrheic keratosis associated
	with malignancy
Loeffler's syndrome	patchy infiltrate of lungs and
	eosinophilia; may complicate
	creeping eruption (larva
	migrans)
Lofgren's syndrome	sarcoid may appear with fever
	polyarthralgias
	uveitis
	bilateral hilar adenopathy
	fatigue
	erythema nodosum
Louis–Barr's syndrome	ataxia-telangiectasia
Maffucci's syndrome	multiple vascular
	malformations with
	dyschondroplasia

MAGIC syndrome | Behçet's disease + relapsing polychondritis
mouth and genital and inflamed cartilage

Mal de Meleda syndrome | stocking-glove distribution of hyperkeratosis
no dental abnormalities

Marinesco–Sjögren syndrome | cerebellar ataxia
mental retardation
congenital cataracts
inability to chew food
thin brittle fingernails
sparse hair

Marshall's syndrome | resembles Sweet's syndrome
but followed by acquired cutis laxa

Melkersson–Rosenthal syndrome | recurring facial paralysis/paresis
soft nonpitting edema of lips
scrotal tongue (plicated tongue)

Menkes' kinky hair syndrome | pili torti, monilethrix, trichorrhexis nodosa
drowsiness, lethargy
convulsive seizures
neurologic deterioration

Michelin Tire Baby syndrome | folded skin with scarring

Moon-boot syndrome | immersion foot (warm-water)

MORFAN syndrome | mental retardation
overgrowth
remarkable face
acanthosis nigricans

Moynahan's (leopard) syndrome	Lentigines
	EKG conduction defects
	Ocular hypertelorism
	Pulmonary stenosis
	Abnormal genitalia
	Retarded growth
	Deafness
Mucocutaneous lymph node syndrome	Kawasaki's disease
Muir–Torre syndrome	sebaceous tumors
	keratoacanthomas
	associated with multiple low-grade tumors
Multiple hamartoma syndrome	Cowden's disease
	trichilemmomas of ears, nose, mouth
	increased risk of thyroid follicular and breast adenocarcinoma
Naegeli–Franceschetti– Jadassohn	reticulate pigmentation
	hypohidrosis
	absent dermatoglyphics
	abnormal teeth with loss
	palmoplantar keratoderma
Nail-patella syndrome	posterior iliac horns
	aplastic / hypoplastic patellae
	nail dystrophy with ulnar sparing

NAME syndrome	nevi
	atrial myxoma
	myxoid neurofibromas
	ephelides
Nelson's syndrome	pituitary MSH-producing tumor
Netherton's sydnrome	ichthyosiform dermatitis
	hair abnormality
	atopic dermatitis
Nicolau syndrome	ischemic pallor following IM injection
Nicolau–Balus syndrome	micropapular eruptive syringomas
	milial cysts
	atrophoderma vermiculata
Nonne–Milroy–Meige syndrome	hereditary lymphedema
Noonan's syndrome	hypertelorism
	prominent ears
	webbed neck
	short stature
	undescended testes
	low post neck hairline
	cardiovascular abnormalities
	cutis valgus
Occipital horn syndrome	variant of Menkes' syndrome
Oculoglandular syndrome of Parinaud	chronic granulomatous conjunctivitis
	preauricular adenopathy

Odonto-tricho-ungual-digital-palmar	natal teeth
	trichodystrophy
	prominent interdigital folds
	simian-like hands with palmar creases
	ungual digital dystrophy
Olmsted syndrome	hyperkeratotic keratoderma in infancy surrounded by erythematous margins
Omenn's syndrome	mimics GVHD
	exfoliative erythroderma at few weeks
	eosinophilia
	diarrhea
	hepatosplenomegaly
	lymphadenopathy
	hypogammaglobulinemia
Oral-ocular-genital syndrome	classic finding of vitamin B2 deficiency
PAPA syndrome	pyogenic arthritis
	pyoderma gangrenosum
	severe cystic acne
Papillon–Lefevre syndrome	palmoplantar hyperkeratosis
	periodontosis
Parry–Romberg syndrome	progressive facial hemiatrophy
	epilepsy
	exophthalmos
	alopecia
Peutz–Jeghers syndrome	lentigines
	GI polyps

PHACE syndrome	posterior fossa malformation (Dandy–Walker)
	hemangiomas
	arterial anomalies
	coarctation of aorta
	cardiac defects
	eye abnormalities
Plummer–Vinson syndrome	spoon nails (koilonychia)
	hemochromatosis
	microcytic anemia
	dysphagia
	glossitis
POEMS (Crow–Fukase) syndrome	polyneuropathy
	organomegaly
	endocrinopathy
	M protein
	skin changes
PURPLE syndrome	painful purpuric ulcers
	reticular pattern of the lower extremities
Ramsay–Hunt syndrome	involvement of facial and auditory nerves from VZV
Red Man Syndrome	secondary to infusion of vancomycin
Refsum's syndrome	ichthyosis
	atypical retinitis pigmentosa
	hypertrophic peripheral neuropathy
	cerebellar ataxia
	nerve deafness
	EKG changes

Reiter's syndrome	urethritis
	conjunctivitis
	arthritis
	keratoderma blennorrhagicum
REM syndrome	reticular erythematous
	mucinous
Richner–Hanhart syndrome	Tyrosinemia I
	hepatic tyrosine
	aminotransferase deficiency
Riley–Day syndrome	familial dysautonomia
Robert's syndrome	facial port-wine stain
	hypomelia
	hypotrichosis
	growth retardation
	cleft lip
Rombo syndrome	multiple basal cell carcinomas
	trichoepitheliomas
	hypotrichosis
	peculiar cyanosis of hands and feet
Ross syndrome	segmental anhidrosis
	tonic pupils
Rothmund–Thomson syndrome	early-onset poikiloderma
	short stature
	sun sensitivity
	bone defects
	hypogonadism
Rowell's syndrome	erythema-like lesions seen in SLE
Rud's syndrome	ichthyosis

	hypogonadism
	small stature
	mental retardation
	epilepsy
	macrocytic anemia
	retinitis pigmentosa
SAPHO syndrome	Synovitis
	acne
	pustulosis
	hyperostosis
	osteitis
Satoyoshi syndrome	progressive, intermittent
	painful muscle spasms
	alopecia universalis
	diarrhea/unusual metabolism
	endocrine disorders
	2° skeletal abnormalities
Schafer–Branauer syndrome	type 3 pachyonychia congenita
	cataracts
Schimmelpenning syndrome	sebaceous nevus and cerebral
	anomalies
	coloboma
	lipodermoid of the conjunctiva
Schnitzler's syndrome	chronic nonpruritic urticaria
	fever of unknown origin
	bone pain
	hyperostosis
	elevated ESR
	macroglobulinemia (IgM)

Schopf syndrome	hydrocystomas of eyelids
	hypotrichosis
	hypodontia
	nail abnormalities
Scleroatrophic syndrome of Huricz	scleroatrophy
	ridging/hypoplasia of nails
	lamellar keratoderma of hands (and soles)
Secretan's syndrome	factitial lymphedema of the hands
Seidlmayer syndrome	acute hemorrhagic edema of infancy
Seip–Lawrence syndrome	acquired total lipodysrtophy
Senear–Usher syndrome	pemphigus erythematosus
Sjögren–Larsson syndrome	ichthyosis
	spastic paralysis
	oligophrenia
	mental retardation
	degenerative retinitis
Sjögren's syndrome	keratoconjunctivitis sicca
	xerostomia
	rheumatoid arthritis
Sneddon's syndrome	livedo reticularis
	cerebrovascular lesion
Stein–Leventhal syndrome	polycystic ovary disease
	hirsutism
	acne (amenorrhea, uterine bleeding, anovulation, obesity, small breasts)
Stewart–Treves syndrome	angiosarcoma S/P mastectomy

Sturge–Weber syndrome	encephalotrigeminal angiomatosis
	nevus flammeus in area of ophthalmic division of CNV
TAR syndrome	congenital thrombocytopenia
	bilateral absence / hypoplasia of radius, port-wine stain
Thibierge–Weissenbach syndrome	CREST syndrome
TORCH syndrome	toxoplasmosis
	rubella
	CMV
	herpes simplex
Touraine-Solente-Gole syndrome	pachydermoperiostosis
	thickening of skin in folds
	accentuation of creases on face and scalp
	clubbing of fingers
	long bone periostosis
Tricho-rhino-phalangeal syndrome	fine and sparse scalp hair
	thin nails
	pear-shaped broad nose
	cone-shaped epiphyses of middle phalanges of some fingers and toes
Turner's syndrome	webbed neck
	low posterior hairline margin
	cubitus valugs
	triangular mouth
	alopecia

	cutis laxa
	cutis hyperelastica
Unna–Thost syndrome	nonepidermolytic hereditary palmoplantar keratoderma
Van Lohuizen's syndrome	cutis marmorata telangiectatica congenita
Vogt–Koyanagi–Harada syndrome	marked bilateral uveitis
	symmetrical vitiligo
	alopecia
	white scalp hair
	poliosis
	dysacousia
Vohwinkel's syndrome	keratoderma hereditaria mutilans
Von Hippel–Lindau syndrome	retinal angioma
	cerebellar medullary
	angioblastic tumor
	pancreatic cysts
	renal tumors/cysts
Waardenburg syndrome	white forelock
	depigmented macules
	unilateral / bilateral deafness
	lateral displacement of inner canthi
	broad nasal root
	heterochromia of iris
Waardenburg-Shah syndrome	type 4 Waardenburg syndrome
	deafness and pigmentary abnormalities + Hirschprung's disease
	defect in SOX10 gene

Well's syndrome	recurrent granulomatous dermatitis with eosinophilia
Werner's syndrome (adult progeria)	short stature
	cataracts
	skin changes
	premature graying and aging
	alopecia
	atrophy of muscles and
	SQ tissues bone atrophy of extremities
Wiskott–Aldrich syndrome	chronic eczematous dermatitis
	recurrent infections
	thrombocytopenic purpura
Wyburn–Mason syndrome	unilateral retinal arteriovenous malformation
	ipsilateral port-wine stain near affected eye
X-linked lymphoproliferative syndrome	inability to control EBV infection
Yellow nail syndrome	primary lymphedema
	associated with yellow nails and pleural effusions

Dermatology
Mnemonics and Lists

Angioid streaks ("EIC Shop")

Ehlers–Danlos syndrome (type VI)

Idiopathic thrombocytopenic purpura

Cowden's disease

Sickle cell disease

Hyperphosphatemia (familial)

Osteogenesis imperfecta

Pseudoxanthoma elasticum / Pagets disease (bone)

Blue sclera ("gins poem")

Goltz syndrome

Incontinentia pigmenti

Steroids

Pseudoxanthoma elasticum

Osteogenesis imperfecta

Ehrlos-Danlos syndrome (type VI)

Marfan's syndrome

Blue lunulae ("warp")

Wilson's disease

Argyria / Antimalarials

Retrovirals

Phenophthalein

Chanarin–Dorfman syndrome ("idle PM")

Ichthyosis

Deafness

Lipids in leukocytes

Eyes (cataracts)

PMNs/ progressive CNS deterioration

Myopathy/Middle East/Mediterranean

Chemotherapy-induced hyperpigmentation

adriamycin → marked hyperpigmentation of nails, skin, tongue

cyclophosphamide → transverse banding of nails, nail pigmentation

bleomycin → transverse nail banding

5-fluorouracil → transverse nail banding

busulfan → diffuse hyperpigmentation – may be photoaccentuated

5-fluorouracil → hyperpigmentation; possible photoaccentuated

bleomycin → flagellate erythema; urticaria; wheal

fluorouracil → serpentine hyperpigmentation overlying veins proximal to infusion

interferon-α → hypertrichosis of eyelashes

CHILD syndrome

Congenital

Hemidysplasia

Icthyosiform erythroderma

Limb **D**efects

Chromoblastomycosis (causes)

Cladosporium carrionii

Fonsecaea compactum

Fonsecaea pedrosoi

Phialophora verrucosa

Rhinocladiella aquaspersa

Churg–Strauss syndrome ("beansap")

Blood

Eosinophilia
Asthma
Neuropathy
Sinus abnormalities
Allergies
Perivascular eosinophils

Conradi-Hunermann syndrome ("Conradi")

Condrodysplasia punctata
Ocular (cataracts)
Nasal root (flat)
Round ichthyosis (ichthyosiform erythroderma in Blaschko's lines)
Alopecia
Defect of peroxisomal enzyme in fibroblasts
Ichthyosis

Cowden's syndrome ("got tuba")

GI polyps
Oral papillomatosis
Thyroid adenomas
Trichilemmomas
Underdeveloped mandible, maxilla, soft palate, uvula
Breast cancer
Acral keratoses

CREST syndrome

Calcinosis cutis
Raynaud's phenomenon
Esophageal dysmotility
Sclerodactyly
Telangiectases

Cytochrome P-450 inducers (general)

Barbiturates	Propanolol
Carbamazepine	Rifampin
Griseofulvin	Theophylline
Omeprazole	Tobacco
Phenytoin	

Cytochrome P-450 inhibitors (general)

Azole antifungals	Isoniazid
Calcium channel blockers	Nonsedating antihistamines
Cimetidine	Protease inhibitors
Ciprofloxacin	SSRIs
Clarithromycin	Valproate
Erythromycin	
Grapefruit juice	

CYP 1A2 inducers and inhibitors

Inducers	Inhibitors
Barbiturates	Azole antifungals
Clarithromycin	Cimetidine
Erythromycin	Ciprofloxacin
Phenytoin	
Rifampin	

CYP 2C9 inducers and inhibitors

Inducers	Inhibitors
Barbiturates	Amiodarone
Carbamazepine	Azole antifungals
Ethanol	Cimetidine

Inducers	Inhibitors
Rifampin	Fluvoxamine
	Omeprazole
	Ritonavir
	Sulfonamides
	Trimethoprim

CYP 2D6 inducers and inhibitors

Inducers	Inhibitors
Carbamazepine	Amiodarone
Isoniazid	Cimetidine
Phenobarbital	Fluoxetine
Phenytoin	Haloperidol
Rifampin	Quinidine
	Ritonavir
	Terbinafine

CYP 3A4 inducers and inhibitors

Inducers	Inhibitors
Carbamazepine	Amiodarone
Ethosuximide	Anticonvulsants
Isoniazid	Calcium channel blockers
Griseofulvin	Cimetidine
Phenobaritol	Clarithromycin
Phenytoin	Erythromycin
Rifampin	Grapefruit juice
	Protease inhibitors
	SSRIs

Dykeratosis congenita ("plans")

Poikiloderma
Leukokeratosis
Anemia (fanconi type)
Nails (nail plate aplasia)
Sister chromatid exchange

Drug-induced systemic lupus erythematosus

Anticonvulsants
Chlorpromazine
Hydralazine
Isoniazid
Methyldopa
Minocycline
Procainamide / Penicillamine / Penicillin / Phenytoin / Propylthiouracil / Practolol / PUVA

Drug-induced systemic cutaneous lupus erythematosus

Aldactone	Hydrochlorothiazide
Azothioprine	Piroxicam
Diltiazem	Sulfonylureas
Glyburide	Terbinafine
Griseofulvin	

Drug-induced lichenoid reactions

Allopurinol	Gold
Antimalarials	Hydrochlorothiazide
Beta-blockers	Metformin
Calcium channel blockers	NSAIDs
Captopril	Phenytoin
Dapsone	Quinidine
D-penicillamine	Simvistatin

Drug-induced linear IgA dermatosis

Amiodarone	Glyburide
Captopril	Phenytoin
Diclofenac	PUVA
Lithium	Vancomycin

Drug-induced pigmentation

Slate gray	Chloroquine	Minocycline
	Hydroxychloroquine	Phenothiazines
Slate blue	Amiodarone	
Blue-gray	Gold	
Yellow	β-carotene	Quinacrine
Red	Clofazamine	
Brown	ACTH	Oral contraceptives
	Bleomycin (flagellate)	Zidovudine

Drug-induced Sweet's syndrome

All-trans retinoic acid
Anticonvulsants
G-CSF
Minocycline
Oral contraceptives
Trimethoprim-sulfamethoxazole

Ectothrix infections

Microsporum audounii
Microsporum canis
Microsporum ferrugineum
Microsporum fulvum
Microsporum gypseum
Trichophyton megninii

Trichophyton mentagrophytes
Triphophyton rubrum
Trichophyton verrucosum

Endothrix infections

Trichophyton tonsurans
Trichophyton schoenlenii
Trichophyton soudenese
Trichophyton violaceum

Fluorescent dermatophytes

Microsporum distortum
Microsporum audouinii
Microsporum canis
Microsporum ferrugineum
Trichophyton schoenlenii
Microsporum gypsum

Focal dermal hypoplasia (Goltz) ("focal")

Female

Osteopathia striata

Colobomata

Absence of dermis

Lobster claw deformity

Green birefringence with polarized light

Amyloid
Colloid milium
Porphyrias
Lipoid proteinosis

Henoch-Schönlein purpura ("hap")

Hematuria
Abdominal pain / **A**rthralgias
Purpura / **P**ain

Hermansky-Pudlak syndrome ("pudlak")

Platelet defect
Ulcerative (granulomatous) colitis
Dyspigmentation (vitiligo)
Lipid in monocytes
Actinic **K**eratoses / **A**canthosis nigricans / **A**typical nevi

HLA associations

Behçet's diseaee	HLA-B51
Dermatitis herpetiformis	HLA-DQw2; B8; DR3
Erythema multiforme	HLA-DQ3
Erythema multiforme (HSV associated)	HLAa-B15
Psoriasis	HLA-Cw6

Kawasaki's disease ("fresca")

Fever
Rash
Edema
Strawberry tongue
Conjunctivitis
Adenopathy

LAMB syndrome

Lentigines
Atrial myxomas
Mucinosis (papular)
Blue nevus

Layers of scalp ("scalp")

Skin

Connective tissue

Aponeurosis

Loose areolar layer

Periosteum

LEOPARD syndrome

Lentigines

EKG abnormalities

Ocular hypertelorism

Pulmonic stenosis

Abnormal genitalia

Retarded growth

Deafness

Lupus Erythematosus, diagnostic criteria

("champions nd")

CNS disorder (seizures/psychosis)

Hematologic disorder

ANA in abnormal titer

Malar erythema

Photosensitivity

Immunologic disorder (+LE-prep; anti-DNA Ab or Sm Ag)

Oral ulcers

Nonerosive arthritis

Serositis (pericarditis/pleurisy

Nephropathy (albuminuria/cellular casts)

Discoid LE

Mast cell degranulators (non-immunologic) ("prom")

Polymyxin B
Radiocontrast dye
Opioids
Muscle relaxants (succinylcholine, tubocurarine)

Mastocytosis types ("mast")

Maculopapular
All over
Solitary nodule
TMEP

Muir-Torre syndrome ("sank")

Sebaceous Adenomas
Neoplasms (visceral)
Keratoacanthomas

NAME syndrome

Nevi
Atrial myxomas
Myxoid neurofibroma
Ephelides

Netherton syndrome

Trichorrhexis invaginata
Hypernatremia
Eczema
Pili torti
Ichthyosis linearis circumflexa
Trichorrhexis nodosa
Seborrhea

Pachyonychia congenita

Nail dystrophy with subungual hyperkeratosis

Follicular hyperkeratosis

Benign leukoplakia

Palmoplantar keratosis

Painful dermal tumors ("bengal")

Blue rubber bleb nevus syndrome

Eccrine spiradenoma

Neuroma / Neurilemmoma

Glomus tumor (solitary) / **G**ranular cell tumor

Angiolipoma / **A**ngioleiomyoma / **A**diposis dolorosa

Leiomyoma

Perforating disorders ("kerrp")

Kyrles' disease

Elastosis perforans serpiginosum

Reactive perforating collagenosis

Perforating folliculitis

Perforating disorder of renal disease and diabetes

POEMS syndrome

Polyneuropathy

Organomegaly

Endocrinopathy

M protein

Skin changes

Puritus without skin rash ("herb mend")

Hepatic disease

Endocrinopathy

Renal disease

Blood dyscrasias

Malignancy

External infestations

Neurosis

Drug-induced

Refsum's syndrome (phytanic acid oxidase deficiency)

Cerebellar ataxia

Retinitis pigmentosa ("salt and pepper" pattern)

Ichthyosis

Polyneuropathy (ataxia, cardiac block, deafness)

Riley-Day syndrome ("didi data")

Deficient lacrimation

Increased sweating

Drooling

Impaired temperature/BP regulation

Decreased pain sensation

Absent tendon reflexes

Transient erythema

Absence of fungiform / circumvallate papillae on tongue

Rombo syndrome ("bath mc")

Basal cell carcinomas

Atrophoderma vermiculata

Trichoepitheliomas

Hypotrichosis

Milia

Cyanosis (acral)

Sarcoid syndromes

Blau's syndrome: micropapules, arthritis, uveitis
Darier–Roussy: subcutaneous nodules of trunk/extremities
Heerfordt–Waldenström: fever, parotid enlargement, facial nerve
Lofgren's: EN, migratory polyarthritis, fever, iritis
Mikulicz's: bilateral sarcoid (parotid, submandibular, lacrimal gland)

Schnitzler's syndrome

chronic, nonpruritic urticaria
fever of unknown origin
disabling bone pain
hyperostosis
increased ESR
macroglobulinemia (usually IgM κ)

Sjögren-Larsson syndrome ("Larson")

Lamellar ichthyosis
Autosomal recessive
Retinitis pigmentosa
Spastic paresis / **S**eizures / **S**parse hair
Ocular defects (glistening macular dots)
NAD oxidoreductase

Wegener's granulomatosis ("rough")

Radiograph (chest)
Oral ulcers
Urinary sediment
Granulomas
Hemoptysis

Wiskott-Aldrich (XLR inheritance) ("tie")

    Thrombocytopenia

    Infections

    Eczema

Vitamins ("the rich never pay cash")

The	Thiamine (B1)
Rich	Riboflavin (B2)
Never	Niacin (B3)
Pay	Pyridoxine (B6)
Cash	Cyanocobalimin (B12)

Dermatopathology Pearls

Big Blue Balls in the Dermis

Cylindroma

Lymphoma

Melanoma

Merkel cell carcinoma

Spiradenoma

"Bodies" in dermatopathology

Arão–Perkins elastic bodies → male pattern alopecia

Asteroid body → sporotrichosis, sarcoidosis, TB, leprosy

Civatte body → lichen planus, lupus erythematosus, GVHD

Councilman body → cytoplasmic inclusions, BCC

Donovan body → granuloma inguinale

Farber body → Farber's disease

Guarnieri body → vaccinia, smallpox

Henderson-Patterson body → molluscum contagiosum

Kamino body → Spitz nevi

Lafora bodies → Lafora disease

Medlar body → chromoblastomycosis

Michaelis–Gutmann body → Malacoplakia

Mulberry cells → hibernoma

Psammoma body → nevocellular nevus, cutaneous meningioma

Russel body → rhinoscleroma; plasmocytosis

Schaumann bodies → sarcoidosis

Verocay body → schwannoma

Weibel–Palade body → endothelial cells

Zebra bodies → Farber's/Fabry's disease

"Busy dermis"

Blue nevus

Dermatofibroma

Kaposi's sarcoma

Granuloma annulare

Metastatic (breast) cancer

Lichen myxedematosus

Necrobiosis lipoidica

Eosinophilic spongiosis ("see a chip")

Spongiotic drug eruption

Erythema toxicum neonatorum

Eosinophilic pustular folliculitis (Ofuji)

Arthropod and Allergic contact

Cutaneous larva migrans

Herpes gestationis and Dermatitis herpetiformis

Incontinentia pigmenti / Infestations

Pemphigus / Pemphigoid

Grenz zone

Granuloma faciale

Leprosy

Erythema elevatum diautinum

Intraepidermal eosinophilic vesicles

Herpes gestationis

Arthropod / Allergic

Pemphigus / Pemphigoid

Incontinentia pigmenti

Erythema toxicum neonatorum / Eosinophilic pustular
folliculitis Ofuji

Non-inflammatory subepidermal blister

Porphyria / variegate porphyria

Epidermolysis bullosa / epidermolysis bullosa acquisita

Suction blister

Coma bullae

Hemodialysis

Bullous diabeticorum

Sweat gland necrosis

Cell-poor pemphigoid

Bullous amyloid

Polymorphous light eruption

Patchy dermal lymphocytic infiltrates ("5 Ls")

Lupus erythematosus

Lymphocytic leukemia

Lymphocytoma cutis

Light (polymorphous) eruption of the plaque type

Lymphocytic infiltration of the skin of Jessner

Parasitized histiocytes

Granuloma inguinale

Rhinoscleroma

Trypanosomiasis / Toxoplasmosis

Leishmaniasis

Histoplasmosis

Pseudocarcinomatous hyperplasia

Blastomycosis

Bromoderma

Chronic ulcer edges (pyoderma gangrenosum, burns, stasis dermatitis, basal cell epithelioma, lupus vulgaris, osteomyelitis, scrofuloderma, gumma, granuloma inguinale)

Granular cell tumor

Hidradenitis suppurativa

Pyoderma vegetans

Squamous cell carcinoma

Subepidermal bullae with neutrophils

Bullous pemphigoid

Bullous lupus erythematosus

EBA

Linear IgA

Dermatitis herpetiformis

NOTES

INDEX